ACE
THE
THINKING SKILLS
ASSESSMENT

The foundation of every state is the education of its youth.
—Diogenes of Sinope

ACE THE THINKING SKILLS ASSESSMENT

Dr Neel Burton
BSc, MBBS, MRCPsych, MA (Phil), AKC

Green Templeton College
University of Oxford, Oxford, UK

A

Acheron Press
Flectere si nequeo superos
Acheronta movebo

© Acheron Press 2014

Published by Acheron Press

A CIP catalogue record for this book is available from the British Library.

ISBN 978 0 9929127 1 0

Typeset by Phoenix Photosetting, Chatham, Kent, United Kingdom
Printed and bound by SRP Limited, Exeter, Devon, United Kingdom

About the Author

Dr Neel Burton is a psychiatrist, philosopher, writer, and wine-lover who lives and teaches in Oxford, England.

Apart from teaching psychiatry at Green Templeton College, Dr Burton teaches courses on entrance examinations such as the TSA, UKCAT, and BMAT, and tutors students on a one-to-one basis.

He is the recipient of the Society of Authors' Richard Asher Prize, the British Medical Association's Young Authors' Award, and the Medical Journalists' Association Open Book Award.

Some of his other books include:

The Meaning of Madness
Hide and Seek: The Psychology of Self-Deception
The Art of Failure: The Anti Self-Help Guide
Plato: Letters to my Son
The Concise Guide to Wine and Blind Tasting

You can find Dr Burton at www.neelburton.com, as well as on Facebook and Twitter.

Contents

CHAPTER 1
Introduction to the TSA

The Thinking Skills Assessment (TSA) was designed, developed, and extensively researched by the Admissions Testing Service. It is used as an admission test for an increasing number of courses at an increasing number of universities—especially those courses, such as PPE (Philosophy, Politics, and Economics) at Oxford, for which thinking and problem-solving skills are critical.

In the TSA, the emphasis is on cognitive (or thinking) skills rather than knowledge as such, and the amount of knowledge required is minimal. The Admissions Testing Service website, which you ought to consult for the most up-to-date information, specifically states that 'students don't need any familiarity with specific texts or theoretical frameworks—they're simply being tested on their ability to think through problems and arguments, critically and logically'. This means that the best way to prepare for the TSA is to develop your thinking skills by working through a large number of TSA-style questions.

You should look at the TSA as an opportunity rather than a hurdle. Most obviously, it is an opportunity to stand out from your competition. From the point of view of academic institutions, the TSA offers an additional selection filter for courses that typically attract a large field of high-achieving applicants. As TSA scores closely correlate with future academic achievement, the TSA provides a valid and objective benchmark against which all applicants can be measured, regardless of background, nationality, gender, qualifications, and other such factors.

But the TSA also presents an opportunity to hone your thinking skills, which are going to be far more important than your actual course content to the impression that you are going to make on the world, to say nothing of your private happiness, which is perhaps the greater and yet more disregarded challenge. As the 20th century American psychologist BF Skinner (he of the rats) once said, 'Education is what survives when what has been learnt has been forgotten.'

Who needs to sit the TSA?

At the time of writing, the TSA is being used by the University of Oxford for certain courses, the University of Cambridge for certain courses in certain colleges, University College London (UCL) for European Social and Political Studies (ESPS), and the University of Leiden in the Netherlands for its International Bachelor of Science in Psychology (IBP) programme.

At Oxford, the TSA is used for the following courses:

- Economics and Management
- Experimental Psychology

- Geography
- Philosophy and Linguistics
- Philosophy, Politics, and Economics (PPE)
- Psychology and Linguistics
- Psychology and Philosophy.

At Cambridge, a significant number of colleges use, or may use, the TSA for the following courses:

- Computer Science
- Economics
- Engineering
- Human, Social, and Political Sciences
- Land Economy
- Natural Sciences.

This information is apt to change, so remember to check the websites of the Admissions Testing Service and of the applicable universities and colleges.

What does the TSA involve?

The TSA is a pen-and-paper test with two sections. Section 1 consists of multiple-choice questions testing problem-solving skills, including numerical and spatial reasoning, and critical thinking skills, including understanding argument and reasoning using everyday language. Section 2 consists of a writing task.

Section 1 is 90 minutes long and comprises 50 multiple-choice questions.

Section 2 is 30 minutes long and you are asked to answer one essay question from a choice of four. The essay questions are not subject-specific.

TSA Oxford and TSA Leiden consist of both sections. TSA Cambridge and TSA UCL consist of Section 1 only.

A version of the TSA that contains only questions testing critical thinking is used for admission to Politics, Psychology & Sociology (PPS) by some colleges of the University of Cambridge.

Again, this information is apt to change, so do check the websites.

Practicalities

TSA Oxford and in general

You must sit the TSA Oxford in the same year that you are applying, regardless of whether you have sat it before or are deferring entry.

The TSA Oxford can be delivered either at your institution or through a global network of open test centres (see the Admissions Testing Service website). Most candidates sit the test at their own school or college. If in any doubt, speak to your Exams Officer or equivalent.

In 2014, test centres can register candidates for the TSA Oxford from 1 September to 17:00 BST on 15 October. You cannot register yourself for the test: your test centre needs to register you. Make sure to obtain from your test centre your candidate number, which serves as confirmation that you have been registered for the test. Some (but by no means all) test centres may charge you an administration fee to cover the costs of running the test.

In 2014, the TSA Oxford takes place on 5 November at 09:00 BST. The scheduled start times for centres outside the UK vary depending on where they are.

On test day, bring a soft pencil (HB or softer) and pencil eraser for Section 1, and a black ink pen for Section 2. For Section 1, enter your answers on the separate answer sheet. For each question, select one of A, B, C, D, or E. If you make a mistake, erase it thoroughly and try again.

Calculators and dictionaries (including bilingual dictionaries) are not allowed. Neither is correction fluid.

Access arrangements are available for candidates with certain conditions such as dyslexia; however, no extra time is allowed for candidates for whom English is not the first language.

TSA Cambridge

In 2014, the TSA Cambridge takes place during the Cambridge interview period. The college you are applying to registers you for the test, free of charge, and informs you of when and where it will take place. The test will take place either at the college itself or at a test centre in Cambridge.

TSA UCL

You normally sit the TSA UCL on an ESPS assessment day at UCL. In 2013/14, these take place on five separate dates from 4 December 2013 to 19 March 2014. UCL registers you and informs you of your TSA test date. There is no cost involved. Arrangements for overseas applicants vary—contact UCL.

TSA Leiden

In 2014, registration for the TSA Leiden opens on 17 March and closes on 28 March. Registration takes place through an online registration system. The entry fee is €100 or £90 or $140. The test takes place on 14 April at the Leiden University Institute of Psychology and at other test centres internationally. On the test day, you need to bring a photo ID—either a passport or national ID card. The results are published on 1 May.

For further and up-to-date details on practicalities, visit the Admissions Testing Service website.

Scoring and results

TSA Oxford and in general

The marking for Section 1 is automated, with each question worth one mark. Your raw score is converted on the TSA scale, which runs roughly from 0 to 100. The TSA scale applies the Rasch statistical technique to factor in the question and overall test difficulty and make scoring comparable across different versions of the test. The typical candidate, who by definition is very able, will score around 60 on the TSA scale; only a few exceptional candidates will score above 80.

For applicants to the University of Oxford, Section 2 is not formally marked. Instead, it is reviewed by the admissions tutor(s) of the Oxford college to which you are applying. For further information on the format and marking of the essay, see Chapter 6.

Results are released at midnight on 15 January via the Results Online system (which only supports Internet Explorer and Firefox browsers). Results are only released to candidates who have applied to one of the courses requiring the TSA at the University of Oxford. To access your results, you will require the PIN that you will have been given on the day of the test.

Your results will be supplied to the Oxford college to which you are applying. The precise role of the results in the selection process varies from one subject to another. For further information, refer to the website of your chosen course.

Remember that the TSA is only one of the elements used in the selection process, alongside academic record, predicted grades, UCAS personal statement, interview performance (if invited), and so forth. In my experience, students tend to underestimate the importance of the personal statement and interview performance.

If you feel that temporary illness, injury, or any other issue affected your test result, you can ask for this to be taken into account as a special consideration. To do so, you need to submit a Special Considerations form within seven days of the test date, together with a covering letter written on the test centre's headed notepaper.

TSA Cambridge

The date on which the results are published varies from college to college. The precise role of the results in the selection process varies. If you wish to ask for special consideration, you need to submit your request directly to the college to which you are applying.

TSA UCL

The Admissions Testing Service releases your results to UCL; it does not release them directly to you. UCL will let you know when the results are due to be released.

TSA Leiden

Results are released on 1 May. For information on the format and marking of the Section 2 essay, see Chapter 6.

For further and up-to-date details on scoring and results, visit the Admissions Testing Service website.

CHAPTER 2
Structure and components of TSA Section 1

The TSA assesses problem solving and critical thinking.

Problem solving involves reasoning using numerical and spatial skills, and tests your ability to find or create a solution to a problem.

Critical thinking involves reasoning using everyday written language, and tests your ability to understand arguments and assess their validity.

Both problem solving and critical thinking are assessed through multiple-choice questions.

Format of the questions

For each multiple-choice question, you are presented with a stimulus, followed by the question itself and five answer options from which to choose. Only one of the five options is correct.

For problem solving questions, the stimulus may include a diagram, a table, or a graph. In some cases, the answer options may correspondingly consist of diagrams or graphs.

For critical thinking questions, the stimulus is a passage of text, often of about 100 words in length.

Distribution of the questions

You have 90 minutes in which to answer a total of 50 questions.

The standard TSA contains 25 problem solving questions and 25 critical thinking questions.

Both question types vary in difficulty from very easy to very hard.

The question types are not strictly separated, so expect to be moving back and forth between problem solving questions and critical thinking questions.

Problem solving questions

The mathematics required for problem solving questions is basic: simple fractions, percentages and percentage operations, calculations in everyday contexts, and such like. A GCSE in mathematics is more than enough to cover you. As you will discover, the real challenge is not so much in the mathematics itself, but in quickly being clear about the numbers and operations required to solve what are, in effect, real life problems.

6

There are, according to the Admissions Testing Service, three types of problem solving question:

- Relevant selection
- Finding procedures
- Identifying similarity.

I distinguish a distinct and important fourth type of question which tests spatial reasoning.

Most questions are clearly of one type or other, but some include elements of more than one type. It seems that only a very small proportion of the questions involves identifying similarity: so small, in fact, that you can almost ignore the type.

Relevant selection involves triaging information, discarding unimportant information, and drawing out the information required to find a solution.

Finding procedures involves manipulating the relevant information to generate a solution. The questions typically involve numerical reasoning with three or four numbers.

Identifying similarity involves selecting a situation with a similar structure to the one with which you are presented.

Spatial reasoning involves visualising problems or examining shapes and patterns from different angles and perspectives.

Don't worry if you are not yet completely clear about what these question types involve.

Critical thinking questions

An argument consists of evidence (or premises), from which a conclusion is drawn. For example:

All dogs are mammals. (Premise 1)
All mammals are animals. (Premise 2)
Therefore, all dogs are animals. (Conclusion)

Obviously, in complex arguments, the premises and the conclusion may be far more difficult to identify. In some cases, arguments may contain an unstated or invalid conclusion, that is, a conclusion that does not derive or follow from the premises. In other cases, arguments may contain hidden assumptions that are in fact integral premises of the argument—assumptions without which the argument falls apart. For example:

Moira is gifted in the arts. She has very good taste.

This argument can be rendered as,

Moira is gifted in the arts. (Premise 1)

People who are gifted in the arts have very good taste. (Hidden assumption)

7

Therefore, Moira has very good taste. (Conclusion)

Note that premises do not have to be true for a conclusion to be valid. In the following example, the conclusion is valid whether or not you believe the premises to be true.

Athos is a courageous man. (Premise 1)
Courageous men are virtuous men. (Premise 2)
Virtuous men are wise men. (Premise 3)
Therefore, Athos is a wise man. (Conclusion)

Your role is *not* to evaluate the truth claims of the premises, but to examine the validity of the argument.

In the TSA, there are seven types of critical thinking question:

- Summarising (or extracting) the main conclusion of a passage.
- Drawing a conclusion from the passage.
- Identifying a hidden assumption in the argument.
- Assessing the impact of additional evidence on the argument's validity.
- Detecting reasoning errors: identifying the flaw in the argument.
- Matching arguments: identifying an argument with the same logical structure as that in the passage.
- Applying principles: identifying a statement that follows the same principle as that relied upon by the argument in the passage.

Again, don't worry if you are not yet completely clear about what these question types involve.

CHAPTER 5
Critical thinking

As discussed in Chapter 2, there are seven types of critical thinking question in the TSA:

- Summarising (or extracting) the main conclusion of a passage.
- Drawing a conclusion from the passage.
- Identifying a hidden assumption in the argument.
- Assessing the impact of additional evidence on the argument's validity.
- Detecting reasoning errors: identifying the flaw in the argument.
- Matching arguments: identifying an argument with the same logical structure as that in the passage.
- Applying principles: identifying a statement that follows the same principle as that relied upon by the argument in the passage.

Before delving into each of these question types, it is worth considering a few points about arguments in general.

Arguments are attempts to persuade by providing reasons (or premises or propositions) in support of a particular claim (or conclusion). In a deductive or 'truth-preserving' argument, the conclusion follows from the premises as their logical consequence; in an inductive argument, the conclusion is merely supported or suggested by the premises.

In many cases, arguments are implicit, meaning that their rational structures and their relationships are not immediately apparent, and need to be made explicit through analysis. In some cases, one element (or several elements) of an argument may appear to be missing because it is implicitly assumed, that is, taken for granted.

Each premise and the conclusion can be either true or false. The argument itself can be either valid or invalid. An argument is valid if and only if the truth of the conclusion is a logical consequence of the premises, regardless of the truth or falsity of the premises. Thus, the following is a valid argument.

All organisms with wings can fly. (Premise 1, False)
Penguins have wings. (Premise 2, True)
Therefore, penguins can fly. (Conclusion, False)

Although the above argument is valid, it is unsound. For an argument to be both valid and sound, all of its premises have to be true. In the TSA, the emphasis is much more on validity or logic than on soundness or truth. For an inductive argument, the equivalent of soundness is cogency. An inductive argument is cogent if its premises are true and they render the truth of the conclusion probable.

When trying to decide whether the logical form of a deductive argument is valid or invalid, it can be useful to formulate a counter example, or counter argument, with exactly the same form, with premises that are true under a given interpretation but a conclusion that is false under that interpretation.

Argument:
Some farmers are landowners.
Some landowners are aristocrats.
Therefore, some farmers are aristocrats.

Counter argument:
Some insects are herbivores.
Some herbivores are mammals.
Therefore, some insects are mammals.

To formulate counter arguments, it can help to summarise the argument in symbol form. Both of the above arguments follow the same (invalid) form:

Some A are B.
Some B are C.
Therefore, some A are C.

Logical fallacies

A logical fallacy is some kind of defect in an argument, and may be unintentional or intentional (with the aim to deceive).

A formal fallacy is an invalid type of argument like the one above: it is a deductive argument with an invalid form, and is invalid irrespective of the content of the argument.

An informal fallacy is an argument that can be identified only through an analysis of the actual content of the argument. Informal fallacies often turn on the misuse of language, for example, using a key term or phrase in an ambiguous way, with one meaning in one part of the argument and another meaning in another part of the argument (fallacy of equivocation). Informal fallacies can also distract from the weakness of the argument, or appeal to the emotions rather than to reason. Informal fallacies are frequently although not exclusively found in inductive arguments, and can be hard to uncover. One way to think about it is that, whereas formal fallacies are invalid, informal fallacies are unsound.

The following non-exhaustive list of formal and informal fallacies should give you a greater insight into bad arguments. When reading through the list—which I think should be rather enjoyable—don't worry about what the fallacies are called. Just focus on how they work—or don't!

False conversion involves switching the subject and predicate terms of a proposition, in a proposition using 'all' or 'some/not'.

> *All wise men are bachelors. Therefore, all bachelors are wise men.*
> *Some books are not novels. Therefore, some novels are not books.*

Exclusive premises is drawing a conclusion from two negative premises. No conclusions can ever be drawn from two negative premises.

> *No politicians are philosophers, and no philosophers are bankers. Therefore, no politicians are bankers.*

Affirming the consequent (converse error) is to infer the converse from the original statement. The argument has the invalid form: If A, then B. B. Therefore A.

> *If I have the flu, then I have a fever. I have a fever. Therefore, I have the flu.*

Denying the antecedent (inverse error) is to infer the inverse from the original statement. The argument has the invalid form: If A, then B. Not A. Therefore, not B.

> *If I were rich, I would be able to be happy. I am not rich. Therefore, I cannot be happy.*

Illicit process of the major term (illicit major) is when the major term is distributed in the conclusion, but not in the major premise. (If all members of the term's class are affected by the proposition, the class is 'distributed'; if not, it is 'undistributed'.) The argument takes the form: All A are B. No C are A. Therefore, no C are B.

> *All psychiatrists are doctors (major term). No surgeons are psychiatrists. Therefore, no surgeons are doctors.*

Illicit minor is when the minor term is distributed in the conclusion, but not in the minor premise. It takes the form: All A are B. All A are C. Therefore, all C are B.

> *All doves are birds. All doves are animals (minor term). Therefore, all animals are birds.*

Analogical fallacy is the assumption that things that are similar in some respect are similar in all respects.

> *Hellebores, snowdrops, and crocuses all flower in early spring. Hellebores are deadly, so snowdrops and crocuses must also be deadly.*

Cum hoc ergo propter hoc ('With this, therefore because of this') is the assumption that because two events occur together or are otherwise correlated, one must have led to the other.

> *Schizophrenia is so common in cannabis users that no one can possibly doubt that smoking cannabis is an important cause of schizophrenia.*

Gambler's fallacy is the false assumption that the outcome of one or more statistically independent events can influence the outcome of another or others.

> *Hailstorms have damaged the vineyards of Burgundy every year for the past three years. So next year is very likely to be a good vintage.*

The runaway train refers to an argument that supports a particular course of action, while also supporting much more of it.

> *We should increase the marginal rate of income tax from 45% to 50% because this will lead to greater income redistribution.*

Begging the question is to argue in circles, supporting the conclusion by means of itself.

> *To allow every man an unbounded freedom of speech must always be, on the whole, advantageous to the State, for it is highly conducive to the interests of the community that each individual should enjoy a liberty perfectly unlimited of expressing his sentiments.*

False precision is to talk about inexact notions in terms of exact numbers.

> *Picasso's 'Boy in Blue' is four times more evocative than Cézanne's 'Mont Sainte-Victoire'.*

> *My house is ten times cosier than yours.*

Genetic fallacy is to reject an argument on the basis of its source or origins.

> *Eugenics is popular with fascists. I could never condone any idea that is popular with fascists.*

Appeal to the popularity is to conclude the truth of a proposition on the grounds that most or many people believe it to be true.

> *Of course he's guilty: even his mother has turned her back on him.*

Argument to moderation is to argue that the moderate or middle view is the right or best one.

> *Some people are in favour of building a third runway at the existing airport, while others are in favour of building a brand new airport. The two parties ought to compromise by erecting a new terminal building at the existing airport.*

Non-anticipation involves rejecting an argument on the basis that it is novel or has been rejected in the past. This is the opposite of the appeal to novelty, whereby an argument is accepted on the basis that it is novel or modern.

> *If congestion pricing is such a good idea, how come it hasn't already been implemented?*

Half-concealed qualification is to hide or gloss over the qualifications that limit the strength of a claim.

> *The B31 iceberg is six times larger than Manhattan, and large enough to warrant special attention from NASA. In November 2013, the giant iceberg broke free from the Pine Island Glacier in Antarctica. This is a fairly unusual place to observe such pieces breaking free from the frozen continent. The area has been closely monitored by researchers who *believe* that global warming *may* be leading to retreat of ice at the landmark.*

Accident is to ignore exceptional cases to bolster or uphold a general rule.

> *I could never become a surgeon. It's wrong to hurt people.*

Bifurcation (false dilemma, false trilemma, etc.) is the presentation of limited alternatives when there are in fact more, giving the impression that the alternatives presented are either mutually exclusive or collectively exhaustive.

You can either come with me or stay at home.

Damning the alternatives is to argue in favour of something by damning its alternatives.

Tim is useless and Bob is a drunk. So I'll marry Jimmy. He's the right man for me.

One-sided argument is to argue for only one side of an argument, while remaining silent on the other side.

It's not worth going on holiday. It's expensive and tiring, and exposes you to all sorts of discomforts and dangers. Besides, by staying at home, you can enjoy your garden and all your favourite foods and entertainments.

Argument from ignorance upholds the truth or falsity of a proposition based on a lack of evidence for or against it.

Despite their best efforts, scientists have never found any evidence of current or past life on Mars. So we can be pretty sure that there has never been any life on Mars.

Ignoratio elenchi (irrelevant conclusion) is to present a valid or invalid argument that fails to address the issue in question. Aristotle asserted that, in a broad sense, all logical fallacies are a form of ignoratio elenchi.

I back military intervention in the Syrian civil war. According to one human rights organisation, at least 150,000 people have so far been killed in the three-year-old civil war, a third of them civilians. Another human rights organisation affirmed that the real toll was likely to be significantly higher at around 220,000 deaths. So you too should back military intervention.

Red herring is the use of irrelevant material to try to bolster an argument.

It would be good for the students if you attended college dinners more often. We have a new chef who trained in a Michelin-starred restaurant. The food is to die for! (OK, so maybe that's not so irrelevant.)

Trivial objections is the use of trivial or frivolous objections which fail to undermine the central argument. Trivial objections is a special form of red herring.

- *Cheating on your wife is immoral.*
- *We got married young. I would like to have more experiences.*
- *That doesn't make it any less wrong.*
- *We haven't been getting on recently. Anyway, she'll never find out.*

Refuting the example involves demolishing the example while leaving the actual argument intact.

- *Politicians are all liars. My local MP promised he would help me, and I haven't heard a word from him since.*
- *That's not true: he sent you a note a few weeks ago.*

21

Summarising the main conclusion of a passage

This type of question involves identifying the main conclusion of a passage, that is, what the author of the passage is really trying to convey. If in any doubt, summarise the argument as concisely as possible. To bring out the logical structure of the argument, try inserting a conjunctive adverb such as 'hence' or 'therefore'. Do not simply assume that the main conclusion is whatever comes last: the main conclusion can be anywhere in the passage, including at the very beginning. Incorrect answer options are often a premise or assumption, an example, a minor conclusion, a partial statement of the conclusion, or an overstatement of the conclusion. Note that a minor conclusion is often recognisable in that it also serves as a premise of the main conclusion. Finally, remember that, if need be, you can test or check the conclusion by working backwards and forwards from the available answer options.

Drawing a conclusion from the passage

With this type of question, the conclusion or main conclusion of the passage is not explicitly stated. Your task is to infer the main conclusion from the passage and then select its closest summary from the list of answer options. To infer the main conclusion, identify and summarise the premises of the argument. Apply conjunctive adverbs like 'so' and 'therefore' to the premises to tease out the main conclusion. Your role is not to assess the truth or falsity of the premises: take them at face value, without bringing in any outside knowledge or wisdom. Get into the skin of the author. What message is he or she trying to convey? What is the point or purpose of the passage? Incorrect answer options are often premises or assumptions, counterpropositions, minor conclusions, and conclusions that are either too specific, too general, or otherwise misguided. Again, remember that you can work forwards as well as backwards from the answer options.

The following is an example of this type of question.

If Emma feels anxious about sitting her exams, choosing a career, taking out a mortgage, marrying her less-than-perfect boyfriend, or indeed anything, then this is because she only has a finite number of opportunities to 'make good'. If she could live forever, she would have an infinite number of opportunities to get things right, and so she could fail as many times as she liked or needed. However, she is only going to live for perhaps another fifty years (some 18,000 days), and that is all the life she is going to have.

Which of the following conclusions is best supported by the above passage?

A. If people could live forever, they would feel even more anxious.
B. If people could live forever, they could fail as many times as they liked or needed.
C. The ultimate cause of all Emma's anxiety is the prospect of her death.
D. We all wish to make a success of our life.
E. Our adult life lasts for about 18,000 days.

According to the passage, if Emma feels anxious about anything, then this is because she only has a finite number of opportunities to 'make good'. This is because she is not going to live forever, that is, because she is going to die. If she were immortal, she would have an infinite number of opportunities to get things right, and so would have no grounds for anxiety. Therefore, the ultimate cause of all her anxiety is death (C). A contradicts the passage. B is a counterproposition offered to the reader, not a conclusion of the passage. However likely D seems, it cannot be inferred from the passage. The final sentence about our life lasting 18,000 days (E) merely serves a rhetorical function (see Chapter 6), underlining the brevity of life for the benefit of the reader. It is not a conclusion of the passage.

Identifying a hidden assumption in the argument

In this case, an assumption is not an explicit supposition or postulation (as in the normal sense of the term), but an implicit, unstated, and therefore hidden premise of the argument, without which the argument struggles or falls apart. Such an assumption is often taken for granted by the author of the passage, and can be simple or subtle, true or false. To identify the assumption, identify the conclusion of the argument and its explicit premises. Summarise the argument by splicing out distracting or cumbersome material. The assumption is the missing premise that zips up the argument. There might be more than one assumption, in which case only one will be contained in the answer options. If you cannot quickly identify the assumption or assumptions, test out each of the options. Incorrect options often contradict the assumption, or they are too general or specific, or they are peripheral to the argument. If an answer option is explicitly stated in the passage it is, by definition, not an assumption.

Assessing the impact of additional evidence on the argument's validity

This type of question asks you to identify the answer option that most strengthens or weakens the argument. Once again, begin by summarising the argument, carving out extraneous material and paring it down to the bare bones. Identify any missing parts of the argument, in particular, any assumptions. Go through every answer option in turn to assess which has the greatest claim to strengthening or weakening the argument. The options often consist of facts that supply or modify an assumption of the argument. Incorrect options may be peripheral to the argument, repeat information already contained in the passage, do the opposite of strengthening or weakening the argument, or strengthen or weaken the argument less than another option.

Detecting reasoning errors: identifying the flaw in the argument

An argument is invalid or flawed if the conclusion is unwarranted by the premises. Begin by summarising the argument. Remember that your task is to assess the validity of the argument, not its soundness. In many cases, the flaw will consist of a misguided assumption or a premise that is not a sufficient or necessary condition for the conclusion, but it could consist of any formal or informal logical fallacy. In some cases, you might need to choose the main or major among several flaws, in which case some of the other answer options will consist of minor flaws.

Matching arguments and applying principles

Matching arguments involves identifying an argument with the same (or a similar) logical structure as that in the passage. In some cases, you may be provided with a passage with a blank space in the argument, and asked to insert the word or phrase that most logically completes the argument. This is often a conjunctive adverb or phrase.

Applying principles involves identifying a statement that illustrates the same principle as that relied upon by the argument in the passage. This might, for example, consist of an ethical or legal principle.

To extract or abstract a logical form or general principle, summarise the argument (where necessary) and examine the relationship between its various components.

Be alert to the presence and function of conjunctive adverbs and phrases. For example, 'furthermore' introduces additional supporting information; 'that said' introduces qualification; 'similarly' introduces comparison; and 'yet' and 'at the same time' introduce contrast.

It might be helpful to sketch out the structure of the argument in symbol form, like so:

If undetermined events such as quantum leaps occur by chance, and if free actions are undetermined events, then free actions also occur by chance.

If all A are B, and all C are A, then all C are B.

In this case, notice that the major and minor premises are universal affirmatives, as is the conclusion. An answer option that does not reflect this structure is going to be incorrect. While the above argument is valid, some of the questions may involve an invalid or fallacious argument.

In many cases, the answer options are quite lengthy, and sifting through them can be quite confusing and time consuming. For applying principles questions, incorrect options may consist of the converse principle, similar but different principles, or mere statements of fact.

As ever, practice is key.

CHAPTER 6
TSA Section 2 (the essay)

TSA Oxford and TSA Leiden consist of both Sections 1 and 2. TSA Cambridge and TSA UCL consist of Section 1 only. Check the Admissions Testing Service website for the most up-to-date information.

Section 2 of the TSA 'tests the ability to organise ideas in a clear and concise manner, and communicate them effectively in writing'.

You have 30 minutes in which to answer one essay question from a choice of four. The essay questions are not subject specific, and do not presuppose a right or wrong answer.

You should write with a black ink pen. Correction fluid is not permitted. Neither is any kind of dictionary.

There is space on the question paper for preliminary notes. Your answer should fit onto the answer sheet, which is lined and two pages (two sides) long. No additional answer sheets may be used.

Candidates with permission to use a word processor must not exceed 1,200 words.

For TSA Leiden, you are given a choice of three questions. Your answer should fit on an answer sheet that is just one page (one side) long. Unlike with TSA Oxford, the essay questions include a certain number of prompters. Candidates with permission to use a word processor must not exceed 550 words.

Marking

For TSA Oxford, Section 2 is reviewed by the admissions tutor or tutors of the Oxford college to which you are applying. It is not formally marked, but is used as qualitative information.

For TSA Leiden, Section 2 is marked independently by two examiners. Each examiner provides two scores, one for quality of content (on a scale of 0 to 5) and one for quality of written English (A, C, or E). The marks of the two examiners are averaged out. However, if there is a large discrepancy between their marks, the essay is marked a third time and checked by the Senior Assessment Manager.

In appraising your essay, tutors and examiners are likely to consider whether you have:

- Defined key terms (where appropriate).
- Rephrased the question or proposition (where appropriate), perhaps so as to precise or limit its scope.
- Explained the importance or implications of the question or proposition.

- Proposed reasonable ways of assessing the competing merits of the propositions or logically resolved their conflict.
- Set out your thoughts clearly.
- Expressed yourself clearly, using concise, compelling, and correct English.
- Applied your general knowledge and opinions appropriately.

Past questions

2013
- Can you ever know whether anyone else has thoughts and feelings like yours?
- Should the supply and use of all drugs be legalised?
- Do countries benefit from immigration?
- How should we evaluate advances in science?

2012
- Should convicted criminals be allowed to vote?
- Does a country's ideal political system depend on its level of economic development?
- Should governments only fund scientific research if it is of direct benefit to society?
- Could a robot ever think like a human?

2011
- Is the general understanding of science damaged by the way it is presented in the media?
- Do patent laws encourage or hinder development?
- Do coalitions necessarily adopt policies which unite party leaders but alienate party followers?
- Should we have a right to choose when and how we die?

2010
- 'Printing and the telephone were truly revolutionary inventions. All the internet brings is a difference in scale.' Is that true?
- Is it justified to insist on facial visibility in public spaces?
- Why do we need banks?
- If two reasonable people claim the same fact as evidence for opposing conclusions, does it follow that it can't actually be evidence for either?

2009
- Albert Einstein wrote that 'The whole of science is nothing more than the refinement of everyday thinking.' Do you agree?
- If 'Humanitarian Intervention' is acceptable, why shouldn't Europe invade the USA to stop it using the death penalty?
- If you can give reasons for your actions, does that mean that your actions are rational?
- What changes in society will follow from increased life expectancy?

2008

(Only three questions)
- When, if ever, is forgiveness wrong?
- Should parking fines be based on the driver's income?
- 'The cause of gender inequality is in the hands of men, but the solution is in the hands of women.' Do you agree?

TSA Oxford specimen paper
- Privacy is only good because people aren't good. In a perfect world we wouldn't need privacy. Is that right?
- In order to be a successful leader, is it better to be loved or feared?
- Is ethical consumerism a solution to poverty, or a dangerous distraction?
- Why is vision so important to human beings?

TSA Leiden specimen paper
- 'Doubt is not a pleasant condition, but certainty is absurd.' —Voltaire
  Explain what this statement means. Argue to the contrary that to be certain about something is not necessarily absurd. To what extent do you agree with Voltaire?
- It is an obscenity that rich people can buy better medical treatment than poor people.
  Explain the argument behind the statement. What assumptions does it make? Argue to the contrary, that patients are entitled to spend money on better healthcare if they choose to do so.
- Science only tells us what is possible, not what is right.
  Explain what this statement means. Argue to the contrary that science helps us to judge what is right. To what extent can decisions about what is right and wrong be informed by science?

Approach

1. Be sure to answer the question very directly.

2. Spend the first few minutes planning and organising your essay on a separate sheet of paper.

3. Have a clear introduction and a conclusion and use transitions to move from the one to the other.

- In your introduction, you might define key terms, rephrase the question or proposition, explain the importance or implications of the question or proposition, and precise or limit the scope or aims of your essay.
- In your conclusion, you might summarise the various aspects of the question or proposition, give your considered opinion, and raise further questions.

4. Examine different aspects of the proposition, especially those you don't agree with!

5. Consider having one or two paragraphs for each aspect. Depending on the question and your approach, a possible structure might be:

- Introduction
- Argument 1
- Argument 2
- Counterargument 1
- Counterargument 2
- Conclusion

6. Prefer quality to quantity. Be clear and concise and avoid repeating yourself. In many cases, a well-structured one-page answer will be more effective than a longer but less cogent essay.

7. Write clearly and legibly. There's no point in being brilliant if no one can read you. If your handwriting is terminally illegible, consider writing in block capitals.

8. Avoid textspeak, slang, and contractions (such as *can't* for *cannot*); at the same time, be careful to avoid pretentious language. When given a choice, almost always prefer the simpler word and the more direct structure.

9. Do not be overly 'scientific': the best or most inspiring writing often includes examples, anecdotes, subtle humour, and emotions. (You can apply this advice to your interview preparation as well.)

10. Do not underestimate the breadth of your general knowledge, or hesitate to display it.

Make sure to practise writing short structured essays. You will find that your writing improves very quickly.

Principles of composition

1. In general, prefer the active voice to the passive voice. 'I will always love you' is much better than 'You will always be loved by me.'

2. Keep or put statements into their positive form. 'She thought that studying Latin was a waste of time' is much better than 'She did not think that studying Latin was a good use of her time'.

3. Prefer simple, direct, and concrete language. 'He grinned as he pocketed the coin' is much better than 'He showed great satisfaction as he took possession of his well-earned reward.'

4. Avoid needless or redundant words and constructions, such as

- The question as to whether (whether)
- In a hasty manner (hastily)
- This is a subject that (this subject)
- The reason why is that (because)
- The fact that I had arrived (my arrival)

5. Keep related words together. 'He noticed a yellow patch right in the centre of his prize lawn' is much better than 'He noticed a yellow patch in his prize lawn that was right in the centre'.

6. Avoid shifts in tense, particularly within a sentence. In general, use the present tense as the base tense as it is simplest and most direct. If you shift out of the base tense, remember to return to it as soon as possible. Similarly, if you address the reader directly as 'you' (recommended), do not then shift to 'one' unless the line could be construed as offensive to the reader.

8. Use variety in sentence length and construction to create variety and rhythm and to emphasise key points. Unless they are masterly, avoid lengthy run-on sentences.

Common errors

1. Apostrophes

Possessive singular

- The apple's core
- The witch's malice
- Charles's friend (not Charles' friend)

Exception for ancient proper names

- Aristotle's *Ethics*
- Socrates' method (not Socrates's method)
- Jesus' resurrection (not Jesus's resurrection)

Do not confuse *its* (possessive pronoun) with *it's* (it is).

2. Commas

Parenthetic expressions

- The burning of the so-called heretics, *often people suffering from psychotic disorders such as schizophrenia and manic-depressive illness*, began in the early Renaissance and reached its peak in the fourteenth and fifteenth centuries.

Before a conjunction introducing an independent clause

- Our position is perilous, but there is still one chance of escape.

Series

- The colours of the Union Jack are blue, red, and white.
- He called the dog, put it on a leash, and left the house.

NB. The second comma in the two above examples is called an Oxford comma, and is optional. It is particularly useful with longer constructions. If you choose to use it (as I do), use it consistently.

3. Semi-colons

Connecting two related but independent clauses

- It is nearly half past five; we cannot reach town before dark.

29

- In many cases, you will be making an educated guess between the two best answer options; in such cases, you will stand a greater than 50% chance of getting it right.
- I had never been there before; besides, it was dark as a tomb.

Don't use semi-colons unless you are confident with their use.

- I had never been there before, and it was dark as a tomb.
- I had never been there before. Besides, it was dark as a tomb.

A few of the examples above are from *The Elements of Style* by Strunk and White, which you might consider reading.

Style guide

Rhetoric is the ancient art of effective or persuasive speaking or writing, especially the exploitation of figures of speech and other compositional techniques (and, some might say, logical fallacies!).

Rhetoric may seem abstract and old-fashioned until you realise that your favourite rhymes and tunes and lines all depend on it for their resonance.

Here, I divide what I consider to be the most effective rhetorical devices into just eight groups.

Although no one expects you to use rhetorical devices in your essay, an awareness of rhetorical devices can lead you to a greater appreciation of the psychology, power, and beauty of language, and so to a greater awareness of your own speaking and writing.

1. Sound repetition

The repetition of a sound or sounds can produce a pleasant sense of harmony, subtly linking or emphasising important words or ideas. There are two major forms of sound repetition: consonance and alliteration. Consonance is the repetition of the same consonant sound. Alliteration is a type of consonance involving the same consonant sound at the beginning of each word or stressed syllable.

And the silken sad uncertain rustling of each purple curtain...
(Edgar Allen Poe)

2. Word repetition

Word repetition can create alliteration, rhythm or continuity, emphasis, connection, and progression.

Words can be repeated in immediate succession (epizeuxis), after one or two intervening words (diacope), or at the beginning and end of a clause or line (epanalepsis).

O dark, dark, dark, amid the blaze of noon...
Bond, James Bond.
The king is dead, long live the king!
Romeo, Romeo, wherefore art thou my Romeo?

A word can also be carried across from one clause or line to the next, with the word that ends one clause or line beginning the next (anadiplosis). This brings out key ideas, as well as their connection, lending the proposition something like the strength and inevitability of hard logic.

> *We also rejoice in our sufferings, because we know that suffering produces*
> *perseverance; perseverance, character; and character, hope. And hope does*
> *not disappoint us.*
> (Romans 5:3)

A word can also be repeated, but with a change of meaning: either a subtle, ambiguous change (ploce) or a more obvious grammatical change (polyptoton). Ploce emphasises a contrast by playing on ambiguity, while polyptoton suggests both a connection and a difference.

> *Love is not love which alters when it alteration finds,*
> *Or bends with the remover to remove.*
> (Shakespeare)

As well as single words, groups of words can be repeated, either at the beginning of successive clauses or lines (anaphora), or at their end (epiphora).

> *I fled Him, down the nights and down the days;*
> *I fled Him, down the arches of the years;*
> *I fled Him, down the labyrinthine ways*
> *Of my own mind...*
> (Francis Thompson)

> *There is no Negro problem. There is no Southern problem. There is no*
> *Northern problem. There is only an American problem.*
> (Lyndon B. Johnson)

If you really want to be flare, you can combine anaphora and epiphora (symploce).

> *When there is talk of hatred, let us stand up and talk against it. When there is talk of*
> *violence, let us stand up and talk against it.*
> (Bill Clinton)

In this particular example, the repetition conveys determination, resolve, and togetherness.

3. Idea or structure repetition

The repetition of an idea or structure can, if used correctly, add richness and resonance to expression. It can also add emphasis; create order, rhythm, and progression; and conjure up a total concept.

Let's start with tautology, which is the repetition of the same idea in a line.

> *With malice toward none, with charity for all.*

Pleonasm is a type of tautology involving the use of more words than is necessary for clear expression.

I am the Alpha and the Omega, the first and the last, the beginning and the end.

The above example is a combination of pleonasm and parallelism. Parallelism is using a similar syntactical structure in a pair or series of related words, clauses, or lines. Three parallel words, clauses, or lines is a tricolon, which is a particularly effective type of isocolon.

Blood, sweat, and tears.

An effective way of emphasising structural parallels is through a structural reversal (chiasmus).

But many that are first shall be last; and the last shall be first.

Do not give what is holy unto dogs, and do not throw your pearls before swine, lest they (the pigs) trample them under their feet, and (the dogs) turn and tear you to pieces.

4. Unusual structure

An unusual structure draws attention and can also create a shift in emphasis.

Hyperbaton is the alteration of the normal order of the words in a sentence, or the separation of words that normally go together. There are several types. Anastrophe is the inversion of ordinary word order. Hypallage is the transference of attributes from their proper subjects to others. Hysteron proteron is the inversion of natural chronology.

Above the seas to stand... (anastrophe)
Angry crowns of kings... (hypallage)
Let us die, and charge into the thick of the fight... (hysteron proteron)

Zeugma is the joining of two or more parts of a sentence with a single verb (or sometimes a noun). Depending on the position of the verb (at the beginning, in the middle, or at the end), a zeugma is either a prozeugma, mesozeugma, or hypozeugma. Here is an example of a mesozeugma.

What a shame is this, that neither hope of reward, nor fear of reproach could any thing move him, neither the persuasion of his friends, nor the love of his country.
(Henry Peacham)

Syllepsis is a type of zeugma in which a single word agrees grammatically with two or more other words, but semantically with only one.

She lowered her standards by raising her glass, her courage, her eyes, and his hopes.
(Flanders and Swann)

A hypozeuxis is the reverse of a zeugma, in which each object is attached to its own verb. The following is also another example of anaphora.

We shall fight on the beaches. We shall fight on the landing grounds. We shall fight in the fields, and in the streets, we shall fight in the hills. We shall never surrender!
(Sir Winston Churchill)

A periodic sentence is one that is not grammatically or semantically complete before the final clause or phrase.

Every breath you take, every move you make, every bond you break, every step you take, I'll be watching you.
(The Police)

5. Language games

Language games such as puns and deliberate mistakes can draw attention to a phrase or idea, or simply raise a smile, by creating new and often ridiculous images and associations. They can also give rise to a vivid image, create ambiguity, and suggest sincerity and even passion.

A pun (or paronomasia) is the use of words with similar sounds, or the use of a word with different senses.

> *Do hotel managers get board with their jobs?*
> *She is nice from far, but far from nice.*

Catachresis is the intentional misuse of a term, applying it to a thing that it does not usually denote.

> *To take arms against a sea of troubles*
> *'Tis deepest winter in Lord Timon's purse*

Anthimeria is the intentional misuse of a word as if it were a member of a different word class, typically a noun for a verb.

> *I'll unhair thy head.*

Enallage is the intentional and effective use of incorrect grammar.

> *Love me tender, love me true.*
> *Let him kiss me with the kisses of his mouth, for thy love is better than wine.*

6. Opposition and contradiction

Opposition and contradiction draws attention, forces thought, can be humorous, and can suggest progression and completion.

An oxymoron is a juxtaposition of words which at first sight seem to be contradictory or incongruous. A paradox is similar, but less compact.

> *Make haste slowly.*
> *What a pity that youth must be wasted on the young.*

Antiphrasis is the use of a word in a context where it means its opposite.

> *A giant of five foot three inches.*

Antithesis is the use of a pair of opposites for contrasting effect. A series of antitheses is a progression.

> *A time to be born, and a time to die; a time to plant, and a time to pluck up that which is planted; a time to kill, and a time to heal…*

7. Circumlocution

Circumlocution or periphrasis essentially works by painting a picture, or conjuring up a complex idea, with just a few well-chosen words.

Hendiadys is the combination of two words, and hendiatris of three.

> *Dieu et mon droit*
> *Sex, drugs, and rock'n'roll*
> *Lock, stock, and barrel*

The latter example is also a merism, which is enumerating the parts to signify the whole. Here's another example.

> *For better for worse, for richer for poorer, in sickness and in health.*

8. Imagery

Obviously, imagery works by conjuring up a particular image.

Metonymy is the naming of a thing or concept by a thing that is closely associated with it.

> *Downing Street*
> *The pen is mightier than the sword.*

Antonomasia, a type of metonymy, is the use of a word or phrase or epithet in place of a proper name.

> *The Divine Teacher (Plato)*
> *The Master of Those Who Know (Aristotle)*

Similar to metonymy, synecdoche is the naming of a thing or concept by one of its parts.

> *A pair of hands*
> *Longshanks (Edward I of England)*

Model essay 1

Should we seek out fame?

To be famous is to be known and recognised. More than that, it is a way of standing out, of being special, of being a 'somebody' rather than a 'nobody' like everybody else. It is also a way of perduring, a way of postponing the inevitable and living on.

Fame is not the only way of living on. A more common and ordinary way of preserving your memory is to have children and, one day hopefully, grandchildren. Compared to fame, children and grandchildren are relatively easy to achieve (animals can do it), but they only preserve your memory for at most three or four generations.

In contrast, leaving behind a significant artistic, intellectual, or social legacy is much harder to achieve, but can preserve your memory for far longer. Some 2,500 years after his time, the ancient philosopher Thales of Miletus continues to be studied by every student of philosophy, but no one remembers the Milesians who mocked him for his poverty.

Even so, a day will surely come when students no longer study Thales, or even Plato (who was the first to distinguish between what he called minor and major immortality)—if only because there are no students left!

For this reason, to search for happiness in immortality, even greater immortality, is never anything more than a vain attempt to delay the inevitable, a subterfuge aimed at fooling yourself that you are a 'somebody' rather than a 'nobody' like everybody else.

More fundamentally, it is to fall into the trap of searching for happiness in an idealised and hypothetical future rather than in an imperfect but actual present in which true happiness is much more likely to be found, albeit with great difficulty.

Of course, this is not to say that you should not seek out individuation and self-realisation—far from it—but only that you should not do so in some vain attempt to secure immortality, or even to secure celebrity, fame, or, better still, honour, within your lifetime.

This also frees you from having to rely on public recognition, which can be just as painful as it can be pleasurable, and which is neither dependable nor indispensable.

Model essay 2

'In the past 60 or 70 years, real term incomes in countries such as the UK and the USA have increased dramatically, but happiness has not kept apace.' Is that true?

In this essay, I shall argue that, far from being happier or just as happy, people today are considerably less happy than people 60 or 70 years ago: they have less time, they are more alone, and so many of their number are on antidepressants that trace quantities of a popular antidepressant have been found in the water supply.

People today have more material comforts and opportunities than ever before. Owing to information technology and other developments, their lives have become much easier. They can afford to work less, often from the comfort of their own homes. They can also look forward to living longer and healthier lives. So why should they not be happier than people 60 or 70 years ago?

Although economists focus on the absolute size of salaries, sociologists argue that the effect of money on happiness results less from the things that money can buy than from comparing one's income to that of others, and in particular to that of one's peers. This is an important part of the explanation as to why people today are no happier than people 60 or 70 years ago: despite being considerably richer and healthier, they have only barely managed to 'keep up with the Joneses'.

But there is more. If I am to believe everything that I see in the media, happiness is to be six foot tall or more and to have bleached teeth and a firm abdomen, all the latest clothes, accessories, and electronics, a picture-perfect partner of the opposite sex who is both a great lover and a terrific friend, an assortment of healthy and happy children, a pet that is neither a stray nor a mongrel, a large house in the right sort of postcode, a second property in an idyllic holiday location, a top-of-the-range car to shuttle back and forth from the one to the other, a clique of 'friends' with whom to have fabulous dinner parties, three or four foreign holidays a year, and a high-impact job that does not detract from any of the above.

There are at least three major problems that I can see with this ideal of happiness. First, it represents a state of affairs that is impossible to attain to and that is therefore in itself an important source of unhappiness.

Second, it is situated in an idealised and hypothetical future rather than an imperfect but actual present in which true happiness is much more likely to be found, albeit with a great amount of hard thinking and soul searching.

Third—and most importantly—it has largely been defined by commercial interests that have absolutely nothing to do with true happiness, which has far more to do with the practice of reason and the peace of mind that this can eventually bring.

Model essay 3

Does true altruism exist?

An act aimed at encouraging or securing the welfare of others is altruistic if, and only if, it is selfless. But can any act ever be entirely selfless?

Even when acts of charity are motivated by nothing but empathy, empathy is always from oneself to another, a sort of projection of the self onto the other. Whenever we empathise with someone's plight, it is because we imagine ourselves in their shoes; the more similar they are to us, the easier it is to imagine ourselves in their shoes and so to empathise with them. And so whenever we are concerned about others, it is really for ourselves that we are concerned.

Conversely, some altruistic acts could be a way for people to escape their problems by occupying themselves with the problems of others. By concentrating on the needs of others, people in altruistic vocations such as medicine or teaching may be able to permanently push their own needs into the background, and so never have to address or even acknowledge them. For this same reason, people who care for a disabled or elderly person may experience profound anxiety and distress when this role is suddenly removed from them.

At the very least, altruistic acts are self-interested because they lead to pleasant feelings of pride and satisfaction, the expectation of honour or reciprocation, or the greater likelihood of a place in heaven; and even if neither of the above, then at least because they relieve unpleasant feelings such as the guilt or shame of not having acted at all.

As I hope to have demonstrated, there can be no such thing as an 'altruistic' act that does not involve some element of self-interest—no such thing, for example, as an altruistic act that does not lead to some degree, no matter how small, of pride or satisfaction. Yet an act should not be written off as selfish or self-motivated simply because it includes some inevitable element of self-interest. The act can still be counted as altruistic if the 'selfish' element was accidental; or, if not accidental, then secondary; or, if neither accidental nor secondary, then undetermining.

In conclusion, while an act cannot be entirely selfless, it can be mostly or primarily selfless, and such an act can be counted as altruistic.

Paper 1

1. All Freezians are Nachters, and all Nachters are Westerians. No Esterian is a Nachter.

    Which of the following is a conclusion that can reliably be drawn from the above argument?

    A   All Nachters are Freezians.

    B   All Westerians are Freezians.

    C   Nachters are sometimes not Westerians.

    D   Freezians are Westerians.

    E   Esterians are never Westerians.

2. *Wuthering Heights* is the best book ever written in the English language. Each year for the past ten years, it has received more votes than any other book in our survey of British readers.

    Which of the following is an underlying assumption of the argument above?

    A   *Wuthering Heights* is the best book ever written in the English language.

    B   Each year for the past ten years, *Wuthering Heights* has received more votes than any other book in a survey of British readers.

    C   Public opinion is a valid indicator of how good a book is.

    D   The public rate books according to how much they enjoyed reading them.

    E   *Wuthering Heights* has a gripping story line and larger-than-life characters.

3. We are investing more money than ever before in our healthcare system, both in absolute terms and as a proportion of our national wealth. That is why life expectancy continues to rise. Today, women are living to an average age of 82.8 years, and men 78.8 years.

    Which of the following states the flaw in the above argument?

    A   Health outcomes in the UK are still poorer than in some other European countries.

    B   Life expectancy could have risen even if there had been no increase in health spending.

    C   Healthier people can expect to live longer.

    D   Life expectancy at birth is also rising.

    E   Despite the increased funding, the healthcare system is sometimes criticised for delivering poor patient care.

4. I live on a country estate. Every six months, my friend Eva comes to stay. John comes every nine months and Allan comes every two years.

All three came in June 2014.

In what month and what year will this happen again?

A June 2020

B June 2018

C June 2022

D September 2017

E September 2019

5. The ninth grade pupils at a school need to choose two out of five different books to read during the summer holidays. The table shows the numbers of pupils taking each book combination.

	Life of Pi	1984	Dubliners	Siddharta
Don Quixote	10	5	6	14
Siddharta	22	15	5	
Dubliners	8	3		
1984	26			

What percentage of pupils reading *Life of Pi* are also reading *Siddharta*? (Give your answer to the nearest percent if necessary.)

A 33%

B 50%

C 52%

D 61%

E 25%

6. The chart shows the turnover of a large company in millions of pounds over a
    period of twelve years.

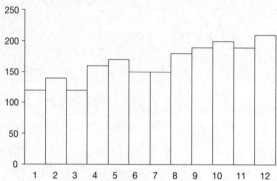

Which of the following graphs shows the annual change in turnover?

A

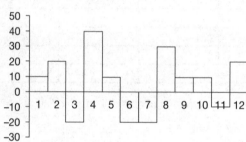

B

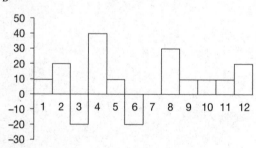

C

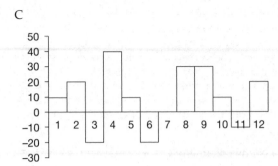

D

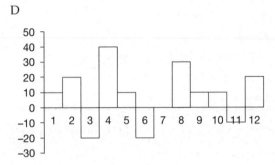

E

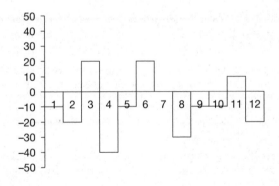

7. For Sartre, people may pretend to themselves that they do not have the freedom to make choices, but they cannot pretend to themselves that they are not themselves, that is, conscious human beings who actually have little or nothing to do with their pragmatic concerns, social roles, and value systems. In pursuing such and such pragmatic concerns or adopting such and such social roles and value systems, a person may pretend to himself that he does not have the freedom to make choices, but to do so is in itself to make a choice, namely, the choice of pretending to himself that he does not have the freedom to make choices.

   Which of the following is a conclusion that can be drawn from the above argument?

   A   The vast majority of people are living a lie.

   B   Self-deception is uncommon.

   C   Man is condemned to make choices, condemned to be free.

   D   People cannot pretend to be other than they truly are.

   E   People are not free to make choices.

8. In some cases, doctor and patient disagree about what constitutes the patient's best interests. In such cases, it is right that the patient's views should prevail. An adult should be entitled to refuse potentially life-saving treatment for whatever reason or no reason at all, so long as the doctor is satisfied that the patient is fully aware of the risks involved in refusing treatment and has not been coerced into refusing treatment.

   Which one of the following best illustrates the principle underlying the above argument?

   A   Every year, many skiers sustain severe and sometimes deadly head injuries. For this reason, skiers should be encouraged to wear helmets at all times.

   B   Cyclists who do not wear a helmet are at greater risk of serious injury. This is why the British Medical Association advocates the compulsory use of helmets.

   C   It is true that some teenagers may be pressurised into taking drugs while not fully aware of the risks involved. But this is a free country, and drugs should be legalised.

   D   The law on wearing seatbelts ought to be repealed. Drivers are well aware of the risks that they are taking if they do not wear a seatbelt.

   E   Yes, Johnny did steal alcohol from the shop; but given that he was coerced into doing so, it would be wrong to punish him.

9. In his influential paper of 1970, tersely entitled *Death*, the philosopher Thomas Nagel asks the question: if death is the permanent end of our existence, is it an evil? Either it is an evil because it deprives us of life, or it is a mere blank because there is no subject left to experience the loss. Thus, if death is an evil, this is not in virtue of any positive attributes that it has, but in virtue of what it deprives us from, namely, life. The bare experience of life is intrinsically valuable, regardless of the balance of its good and bad elements.

   Which one of the following summarises the conclusion of the argument above?

   A   The bare experience of life is intrinsically valuable.

   B   Death is an evil because it is the permanent end of our existence.

   C   Either death is an evil or it is a mere blank.

   D   If death is an evil, this is not in virtue of any positive attributes that it has.

   E   If death is an evil, this is in virtue of what it deprives us from, namely life.

10. The figure shows the basic dimensions of George's basement.

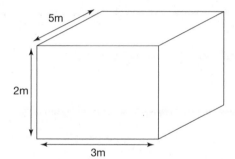

   George would like to convert the basement into a wine cellar. He wants to line one long wall with wine racks. The rack is a modular system, with each module 85cm in height and 120cm in length and containing up to 72 bottles.

   How many bottles can George store in the racks if he lines the wall with as many racks as possible?

   A   72

   B   144

   C   288

   D   576

   E   706

11. The following table shows the pricing scheme for Chatafone Pay as U Call.

Chatafone Pay as U Call Cost of phone: £99			
Cost of calls per minute	£5 voucher	£10 voucher	£50 voucher
Peak	50p	40p	25p
Off-peak	20p	10p	5p

Josefin estimates that she will use 10 minutes peak and 30 minutes off-peak in phone calls per day.

Ignoring the cost of the phone, how much will it cost her in calls over a period of one month (30 days) if she buys only £10 vouchers?

A £7

B £120

C £210

D £309

E £330

12. Various shapes can be created by overlapping two transparent triangles, for example, as in this case, a hexagon.

Which of the following shapes cannot be created by overlapping the two transparent triangles?

A

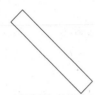

B

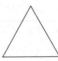

C

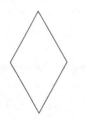

D

E

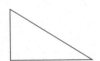

45

13. The Chardonnay grape variety has a 'neutral' or 'malleable' profile, and is sometimes compared to a mirror that reflects the climate and the soil of the region in which it is grown. It is more widespread than any other grape variety, ranging from cool regions such as Chablis in northern France to very hot regions such as South Australia. For these reasons, it is very difficult to generalise about Chardonnay wines. Two Chardonnay wines can have strikingly little in common. For example, Chardonnay from Chablis is typically high in acidity, lean, minerally, and unoaked, whereas Chardonnay from South Australia is big and blousy, with notes of tropical fruits, a full body, high alcohol, and obvious oak influence.

Which one of the following best expresses the main conclusion of the passage above?

A   It is difficult to generalise about Chardonnay wines.

B   Two Chardonnay wines can have strikingly little in common.

C   Chardonnay is more widespread than any other grape variety.

D   Chardonnay is a very successful grape variety.

E   Chardonnay from Chablis is nothing like Chardonnay from South Australia.

14. The layered rocks on Mars seem to have formed under water. They appear to be sandstones, but with a lot of minerals that form when brine evaporates. Calculations suggest that the waters they formed would have been highly acidic. That is bad enough for those who imagine them brim-full of bacteria. But they would also have been highly osmotic. The dissolved chemicals within them would have locked up the water so that it could not take part in biochemical reactions. The 'water activity' of a solution is a measure of the degree to which water is locked up by solutes. Pure water has an activity of 1.0. Seawater's activity is 0.98. The water of primeval Mars was probably between 0.78 and 0.86, and may sometimes have been as low as 0.5.

Which of the following is a conclusion that can be drawn from the above passage?

A   More studies of Martian geology are called for.

B   The calculations need to be verified.

C   Assuming the calculations are correct, life is unlikely to have developed on Mars.

D   The 'water activity' of a solution is a measure of the degree to which water is locked up by solutes.

E   There is, or once was, water on Mars.

15. European history has demonstrated time and again that communism and fascism are doomed to failure. Though based on very different political ideologies, they have both led to large-scale death and destruction and proven to be unsustainable. In light of this, there can be little doubt that parliamentary democracy is the best form of government.

Which of the following most closely parallels the reasoning in the above argument?

A   There are 20 teams in the football Premier League. While Arsenal, Chelsea, and Liverpool are doing very badly, some of the teams are doing very well. Among those teams is Manchester United. I support Manchester United.

B   There are 20 teams in the football Premier League. So far, Manchester United has scored more goals than any other team. In light of this, there can be little doubt that Manchester United is the best team.

C   Look at the Arsenal, Chelsea, and Liverpool football teams. They are all doing very badly. If they go on doing this badly, they will drop out of the Premier League. It should be obvious to their supporters that Manchester United is by far the best team. I support Manchester United.

D   The Arsenal, Chelsea, and Liverpool football teams are all doing very badly. Though the teams have some great players, the players don't work well together and don't score many goals. If the teams go on doing this badly, they will drop out of the Premier League. Manchester United has scored more goals than Arsenal, Chelsea, and Liverpool put together.

E   Arsenal, Chelsea, and Liverpool are very different teams. Yet, all three teams have been doing very badly and have dropped out of the Premier League. To remain in the Premier League, a team needs strong players and a good overall strategy.

16. Jack and Jill live 6 miles apart.

Jack sets off on his motorbike to meet Jill, travelling at a steady 20mph. At the same time, Jill sets off on foot to meet Jack, walking at a steady 4mph.

How long will it be before they meet?

A   10 minutes

B   15 minutes

C   18 minutes

D   20 minutes

E   25 minutes

17. The chart summarises the flying distances between London, Geneva, Moscow, and Hong Kong.

London			
750	Geneva		
2400	2200	Moscow	
10000	9500	7000	Hong Kong

All distances are in kilometres

An aircraft flies from London to Moscow at an average speed of 500 miles per hour (1 mile = 1.6km).

The approximate time taken in minutes is

A   240

B   525

C   180

D   288

E   150

18. Oxford is west of Thame, which is west of Aylesbury.

High Wycombe is east of Thame, and west of Beaconsfield.

Therefore Beaconsfield must be east of

A   Thame, but not necessarily Oxford or Aylesbury.

B   Aylesbury, but not necessarily Oxford or Thame.

C   Oxford and Thame, but not necessarily Aylesbury.

D   Oxford and Aylesbury, but not necessarily Thame.

E   Oxford, Aylesbury, and High Wycombe.

19. As it is, most academics are involved both in research and in teaching. It would be a good idea to separate these functions, with some academics dedicated solely to research and some solely to teaching. Research academics would then be free to focus on research, and teaching academics on teaching, leading to better research and better teaching.

Which one of the following best describes the flaw in the above argument?

A   It considers that research is more important than teaching.

B   It ignores the possibility that research and teaching are mutually reinforcing activities.

C   It assumes that specialisation leads to increased productivity.

D   It fails to recognise that most academics have little interest in teaching.

E   It neglects that, in future, most teaching will take place online.

20. It seems that what makes you a person depends causally upon the existence of your brain, but at the same time amounts to something more than just your brain. What this might be is unclear, and perhaps for a reason. As human beings, we have a tendency to think of our personhood as something concrete and tangible, something that exists 'out there' in the real world and therefore extends through time. _____ it is possible that personhood is nothing more than a product of our minds, merely a convenient concept or schema that enables us to relate our present self with our past, future, and conditional selves.

Which of the following phrases, inserted in the blank space, most logically completes the above argument?

A   However,

B   This being the case,

C   At the same time,

D   Nevertheless,

E   In contrast,

21. Anything that is good is so by virtue of the immediate or deferred pleasure that it can procure. The behaviour of infants confirms that human beings instinctively pursue pleasure and that all of their actions are ultimately aimed at obtaining pleasure for themselves. Just as human beings can immediately feel that something is hot or cold, colourful or dull, so they can immediately feel that something is pleasurable or painful. However, not everything that is pleasurable ought to be pursued. Instead, a kind of 'hedonistic calculus' ought to be applied to determine which things are most likely to result in the greatest pleasure over time, and it is above all this hedonistic calculus that people are unable to handle.

Which of the following is an underlying assumption of the argument above?

A   Human beings can immediately feel that something is pleasurable.

B   The pursuit of pleasure is instinctive.

C   Pleasure is the highest good.

D   Human beings are selfish.

E   People are stupid.

22. The table is representative of people who recently moved house.

		Current house			
		≤ 2 bed	3 bed	≥ 4 bed	Total
Previous house	≤ 2 Bed	200	160	40	400
	3 Bed	80	200	80	360
	≥ 4 Bed	20	120	100	240
	Total	300	480	220	

What percentage of people moved into a larger house?

A   12%

B   26%

C   24%

D   28%

E   30%

23. 12 teams participate in a football tournament.

The teams are divided into two groups of six teams. Each team plays every other team in its group twice, and every other team once.

How many matches are there in total?

A   67

B   91

C   96

D   97

E   109

24. I have 20 coins worth £1.35, and I only have 5p and 10p coins.

How many 5p coins do I have?

A   11

B   12

C   13

D   14

E   15

25. Law school is expensive, time-consuming, and demanding. Instead of going to law school, you should start your own business. By starting your own business, you will get a much better financial return on your money, time, and energy. After three years of building your own business, you will have picked up an invaluable education in how to make money. And if you're successful, you won't ever have to ask someone for a job again.

Which of the following, if true, would most weaken the above argument?

A   Most people believe that it is easier to suffer silently than to think creatively.

B   Most people are frightened of failure.

C   Many new businesses fail.

D   Most people who go to law school do so because they are genuinely interested in the law.

E   A large minority of people who go to law school end up starting their own business.

26. Death, no matter how inevitable, is an abrupt cancellation of indefinitely extensive goods. Given the sheer pain of this conclusion, it is hardly surprising that philosophers throughout the ages have sought, more or less unsuccessfully, to undermine it. Death not only deprives us of life, but also compels us to spend the life that it deprives us from in the mostly unconscious fear of this deprivation. And it is this unconscious fear that holds us back from exercising choice and freedom.

Which of the following best summarises the conclusion of the argument above?

A   Death is an evil because it deprives us of life.

B   Death, no matter how inevitable, is an abrupt cancellation of indefinitely extensive goods.

C   Death is an evil not only because it deprives us of life, but also because it mars whatever little life we do have.

D   Our fear of death is mostly unconscious.

E   If we were not so frightened of death, we would be better able to exercise choice and freedom.

27. Lawyers in Macondo can work as solicitors, as barristers, or both. 32% of lawyers in Macondo work, at least some of the time, as barristers.

Which of the following conclusions can reliably be drawn from the above passage?

1.   More lawyers work as solicitors than as barristers.

2.   Some lawyers work only as barristers.

3.   Some lawyers spend more time working as barristers than as solicitors.

A   1 only.

B   1 and 2.

C   2 and 3.

D   1, 2, and 3.

E   3 only.

28. A farmer has an underground cistern which he decides to calibrate by adding known volumes of water and measuring the depth using a dipstick. His calibration graph is shown below. The horizontal cross-section of the tank is circular at all points.

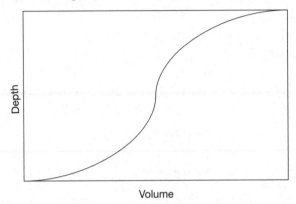

Which one of the following shows the most likely cross-sectional shape of the tank?

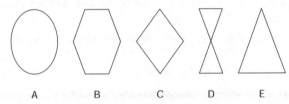

29. Linda bought some shares in X Corp for £5,000. A year later, she sold the shares for a 20% profit.

Three months later, she noticed that shares in X Corp had fallen by 15%. Considering them to be cheap, she decided to reinvest the proceeds of the sale into the shares.

Three years later, the shares had risen by 45% from when she bought them the second time. So she decided to sell them again.

How much profit did she make on her initial investment when she sold the shares for the second time?

A 74%

B 50%

C 45%

D 65%

E 70%

30. A survey of 6th formers at one school found that 30% did not go away on holiday, 25% went on holiday within the UK, and 20% went on holiday in Europe.

Of the remaining people in the sample, 8 went to Asia, 6 went to the USA, and 5 went elsewhere.

How many people participated in the survey?

A   19

B   100

C   75

D   76

E   84

31. There are many novels with a tight plot that have done very badly, in some cases selling fewer than 100 copies. At the same time, a number of very loosely plotted novels—one might almost call them rambling—have risen to become international bestsellers. One in particular has even been adapted into a multi-season television series. So if writers want their novels to be successful, they should plot them very loosely.

Which one of the following is the best expression of the flaw in the above argument?

A   Some writers prefer writing tightly plotted novels.

B   Popularity is not the best measure of the success or failure of a novel.

C   Many loosely plotted novels did not rise to become international bestsellers.

D   Not all novels with a tight plot did very badly.

E   The tightness or otherwise of the plot need not be the factor that determines the success of a novel.

32. If undetermined events such as quantum leaps occur by chance, and if free actions are undetermined events, then free actions also occur by chance.

    Which of the following most closely parallels the reasoning in the above argument?

    A   The bird in the tree is a robin. All robins are orange-breasted. Therefore, the bird in the tree is orange-breasted.

    B   The birds in the tree are robins. All robins are orange-breasted. Therefore, the birds in the tree are orange-breasted.

    C   All mammals are animals. All dogs are mammals. Therefore, all dogs are animals.

    D   All mammals are animals. All animals are forms of life. Therefore, all mammals are forms of life.

    E   All dogs are mammals. All mammals are animals. Therefore, all dogs are animals.

33. The ancient philosopher Protagoras once took on a pupil, Euathlus, on the understanding that he would be paid once Euathlus had won his first court case. However, Euathlus never won a case, and Protagoras eventually sued him for non-payment. Protagoras argued that if he won the case he would be paid, and if Euathlus won the case, he would still be paid, because Euathlus would have won a case.

    Which one of the following is the best statement of the flaw in the above argument?

    A   Under the terms of the original contract, Euathlus was not under any obligation to win a case or even to practice law.

    B   If Euathlus engaged a lawyer to represent him and lost the case, he could claim that it was the lawyer, and not him, who lost the case.

    C   If Euathlus won the case, Protagoras would be liable for the court fees.

    D   Protagoras could not possibly win the case.

    E   If Euathlus won the case, Protagoras would be staking his claim on an event that had not yet taken place at the time of his claim.

34. An airplane flight crew starts its day in Zürich and does two round trips to Madrid in the day. On each arrival at an airport, they take the next scheduled flight back. The timetable is shown below (Zürich and Madrid are in the same time zone).

Zürich—Madrid		Madrid—Zürich	
Depart	Arrive	Depart	Arrive
07:15	09:15	06:30	08:30
10:00	12:00	10:15	12:15
14:30	16:30	17:20	19:20
20:30	22:30	19:50	21:50

How long is it from take-off on their first flight to landing on their last flight of the day?

A   4h 00min

B   10h 05min

C   11h 30min

D   12h 05min

E   15h 35min

35. John is playing a dice game with a triangular die (a die with only three sides). One side scores 1 point, another side scores 3 points, and the third side scores 5 points. John throws the die four times and sums up his score.

Which of the following could **not** be his total score?

A   10

B   12

C   14

D   15

E   18

36. A first aid kit consists of:

- – 1 guidance leaflet
- – 20 washproof plasters
- – 4 triangular bandages
- – 6 safety pins
- – 8 sterile dressings
- – 10 moist wipes

The manufacturer of the first aid kit has all the component parts manufactured separately and then shipped to a warehouse, where the parts are assembled and dispatched to retailers in cartons of 12 complete first aid kits.

In the warehouse, there are: 200 guidance leaflets, 2,000 washproof plasters, 600 triangular bandages, 1,500 safety pins, 3,000 sterile dressings, and 1,200 moist wipes.

What is the maximum number of cartons that can be dispatched from the warehouse?

A   8

B   9

C   10

D   25

E   30

37. The world's population is growing much too fast. Only a dramatic expansion in family planning options in developing countries can quickly and effectively curb population growth. It is often said that there are more people alive today than have ever lived. Whether this is true or not, population growth is threatening people and planet alike with environmental degradation and resource shortages. The increasing frequency of severe weather is evidence that the Earth's climate is changing. Add to that the hole in the ozone layer, melting ice caps, the pollution and depletion of our oceans, desertification, and the increasing rate of species extinction, and it is obvious that we are on the brink of an environmental disaster.

Which of the following is a conclusion that can be drawn from the above passage?

A   It is impossible to avert the environmental disaster to which population growth is leading us.

B   Expanding family planning options is relatively cheap.

C   Only a dramatic expansion in family planning options in developing countries can curb population growth and thereby avert environmental disaster.

D   Population growth is threatening people and planet alike with environmental degradation and resource shortages.

E   There is mounting evidence that we are on the brink of an environmental disaster.

38. The man who is willing to hold out in battle in the knowledge that he is in a stronger position is commonly held to be less courageous than the man in the opposite camp who is willing to hold out nonetheless. Yet, the second man's behaviour is more foolish, and foolish behaviour is both disgraceful and harmful, and so opposed to courage. In the Trojan War, Aeneas often took to fleeing on horses, yet Homer [the author of the Iliad, which is about the Trojan War] praised him for his knowledge of fear and called him the 'counsellor of fear'. This suggests that courage amounts not to blind recklessness, but to the knowledge of the fearful and hopeful in war, and, indeed, in every other sphere or situation. Our use of language supports this idea in so far as children and animals, because they have no sense, are never called courageous but at most fearless.

Which of the following is an underlying assumption of the argument above?

A   Whatever people think must be wrong.

B   Courage is always a fine and noble thing.

C   Children and animals have no sense.

D   Homer can only be right.

E   Courage is a form of knowledge.

39. A recent study carried out by Santosa and colleagues found that people with bipolar disorder and creative discipline controls scored significantly more highly than healthy non-creative discipline controls on a measure of creativity called the Barron-Welsh Art Scale. In a related study, the same authors sought to identify temperamental traits that people with bipolar disorder and creative people have in common. They found that both shared tendencies for mild elation and depression with gradual shifts from one to the other, openness, irritability, and neuroticism (roughly speaking, a combination of anxiety and perfectionism).

Which of the following conclusions is best supported by the above passage?

A   Bipolar disorder predisposes to creativity.

B   Creativity predisposes to bipolar disorder.

C   There is an association between bipolar disorder and creativity.

D   Creative types all have similar temperaments.

E   Not all people with bipolar disorder are creative.

40. The table shows the mock and actual exam results for the final unit of the Wine Diploma.

		Actual exam results	
		Pass	Fail
Mock exam results	Pass	110	10
	Fail	50	70

What percentage of candidates had their results correctly predicted by their mock examination results?

A   50%

B   60%

C   71%

D   75%

E   81%

41. What is the angle between the hour and minute hand of an analogue clock when it is a quarter past three?

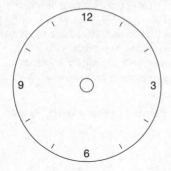

A   0°

B   3.5°

C   5°

D   6.5°

E   7.5°

42. People who smoke cannabis have a 2.5 relative risk of developing schizophrenia. Thus, it is clear that smoking cannabis increases the risk of developing schizophrenia.

Which one of the following, if true, would most weaken the above argument?

A   People who use other drugs also have an increased risk of developing schizophrenia.

B   Many people who smoke cannabis heavily do not develop schizophrenia.

C   People who have never smoked cannabis also develop schizophrenia.

D   People who smoke cannabis have an increased risk of developing other mental disorder as well.

E   A genetic predisposition to schizophrenia is linked to a predisposition to smoking cannabis.

43. People who have suffered from traumatic early life experiences such as parental loss or neglect or emotional, physical, or sexual abuse may be left with intense feelings of despair, helplessness, and worthlessness. Later in life, they may seek out achievement and success as a means of compensating for such feelings. For example, they may wish to be recognised by strangers because they were not recognised by their parents, and they may wish to have control over other people because they had none when they needed it most.

Which of the following, if true, would most strengthen the above argument?

A   Most people who have suffered from traumatic early life experiences have no memory of the trauma.

B   Most people who have suffered from traumatic early life experiences do not seek out achievement and success in later life.

C   Many people who seek out achievement and success in later life did not suffer traumatic early life experiences.

D   Studies have found an association between above average achievement and success and low self-esteem.

E   Studies have found an association between above average achievement and success and traumatic early life experiences.

44. John, Andrew, Mary, and Anne went on a special diet.

At the beginning of the year, they weighed 75kg, 85kg, 80kg, and 70kg respectively.

During the year, they all changed weight by at least 5kg. John lost more weight than either Mary or Anne, while Andrew gained weight.

Which one of the following is not a possible increasing order of their weights at the end of the year?

A   Anne, John, Mary, Andrew

B   John, Mary, Anne, Andrew

C   John, Anne, Mary, Andrew

D   Mary, John, Anne, Andrew

E   Anne, John, Andrew, Mary

45. Before sowing various seeds into a flowerbed, James constructs a wire grid to help him with their layout.

How many perfect squares can be counted?

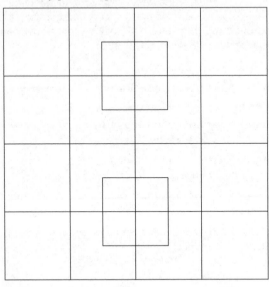

A   26

B   27

C   30

D   39

E   40

46. Schopenhauer draws a distinction between the world of appearances, or 'representation', and the world as it is actually. The world of appearances is the world that we perceive through our senses, and it is governed by certain structures, notably, space, time, and causality. It is our experiencing selves that impose these structures onto the world of appearances, and it is through these structures that we apprehend the individual material things that make up the world as we know it.

Which of the following conclusions is best supported by the above passage?

A   The world as it appears to us is a product of the kind of organism that we are.

B   Individual material things do not exist.

C   Our experiencing self is itself an object in the world of appearances.

D   The world as it is actually is unknowable.

E   Our senses can be mistaken.

47. We should reject the idea that it is just to repay what is owed. Suppose a person lends you a weapon, and, when you prepare to return it, you discover that this person has gone insane. Surely, in such circumstances, it cannot be right to return the weapon to its owner.

Which of the following states the flaw in the above argument?

A   It employs an exceptional case to reject a general rule.

B   It introduces irrelevant material to divert attention from the point being made.

C   It is supported by its own conclusion.

D   You could return the weapon at a later time.

E   You could remove the ammunition before returning the weapon.

48. Krishna works for an insurance company. He has been asked to run a prevention campaign in the month which costs the company most in insurance claims.

To decide when to run the prevention campaign, Krishna examines the statistics for the past ten years and derives monthly averages.

Bearing in mind that a house burglary costs ten times more than a car burglary, which in turn costs ten times more than a theft, in which month should he run the campaign?

	Theft	Car burglary	House burglary	Total #
January	230	60	30	320
February	240	62	28	330
March	255	70	28	353
April	310	75	24	409
May	365	80	20	465
June	450	60	16	526
July	500	50	10	560
August	522	50	22	594
September	350	65	14	429
October	320	70	22	412
November	236	70	24	330
December	250	60	30	340

A   January

B   February

C   August

D   November

E   December

49. With £100, I can buy one atlas and two textbooks.

With £275, I can buy two atlases and seven textbooks.

Which of the following statements is false?

A   Two atlases and three textbooks cost £175.

B   £40 is not sufficient to buy an atlas.

C   £30 is sufficient to buy a textbook.

D   An atlas costs twice as much as a textbook.

E   Three atlases and two textbooks cost £250.

50. A man drives out to work. He leaves his town at a slow speed. Once out of town, he speeds up until he hits some road works, which slow him down considerably. Things get worse, and he grinds to a halt for several minutes. He starts losing patience, and decides to turn round and go back home. This time, the traffic is flowing freely.

Which one of the following graphs best represents the man's distance from home throughout his journey? Distance is represented on the y axis, time on the x axis.

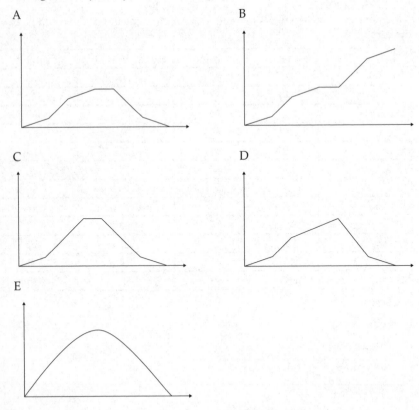

Paper 2

1. Not only is American military equipment better; American troops, unlike China's, have lots of experience of using it in battle. Chinese commanders talk about not being able to match American hard power until 2050 at the earliest. Unlike China and Russia, who have few real friends, America has allies everywhere. That forces America to spread its forces widely and thinly. But history suggests that countries with allies tend to beat those without.

   Which of the following conclusions is best supported by the above passage?

   A   American forces are very well equipped.

   B   After 2050, China will become the dominant power.

   C   China and Russia are allies.

   D   America and China are enemies.

   E   America will remain the dominant power for the foreseeable future.

2. A study of 15 overweight women found that each woman experienced significant weight loss after replacing her normal evening meal with a fruit course. For two weeks, each woman kept to her normal diet other than replacing her evening meal with a fruit course. After taking 20 minutes exercise, each woman was entitled to eat as many fruits as desired, of whatever type. After just two weeks, every woman had lost at least four pounds and, in one case, up to 11 pounds. Interestingly, those who ate more than five pieces of fruit appeared to lose more weight than those who ate five or fewer. Despite its small size, this study suggests that replacing the evening meal with a fruit course is a simple and effective way of losing weight.

   Which of the following, if true, would most strengthen the above argument?

   A   The women adhered strictly to the rules of the study.

   B   The women were highly motivated to lose weight.

   C   The women hardly ate any fruits before they entered the study.

   D   The women exercised regularly before they entered the study.

   E   The women were only slightly overweight before they entered the study.

3. Of 100 students graduating from medical school, 50 are male and 50 are female.

    70 are going straight into house jobs, 20 are going into research posts, and 10 are leaving for others jobs.

    85 are home students, and 15 are international students.

    What is the smallest possible number of male students who are going straight into house jobs and who are home students?

    A   5

    B   10

    C   15

    D   20

    E   8

4. In a particular year, the month of July (which has 31 days) contains five Mondays.

    Which one of the following could not be true?

    A   The 1st of July is a Monday.

    B   The 1st of July is a Saturday.

    C   There are five Saturdays.

    D   There are five Wednesdays.

    E   The 3rd of July is a Friday.

5. The diagram shows the positions of three treasure hunters—William, Krishna, and Eve—on a map, with each square on the map representing one square kilometre. William is at (x, y) $(8, 2)$, Krishna at $(5,5)$, and Eve at $(9,5)$.

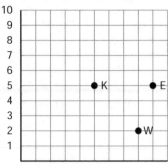

Each of the treasure hunters has carried out a great deal of research on the whereabouts of the treasure. Neither is within 1km of the treasure. However, William knows that he is within 2km of the treasure; Krishna that he is within 3km; and Eve that she is within 3km.

At which one of the following grid points could the treasure be located?

A $(6, 7)$

B $(7, 5)$

C $(7, 3)$

D $(8, 1)$

E $(8, 5)$

6. Most of the time, a person's actions and the neurological activity that they result from are determined by past events and the cumulative effects of those past events on that person's patterns of thinking. Most of the time, a person's actions are determined by a complex amalgamation of addictions, phobias, obsessions, enculturation, socialisation, learnt behaviour, and so on. However, on certain occasions, such as when the person is genuinely torn between two competing and potentially life-changing choices, the degree of indeterminacy in his or her brain rises to such a high level as to permit an undetermined action. Such a 'window of freedom' is more or less uncommon, but can exert a profound effect on all subsequent determined and undetermined actions.

Which of the following best expresses the main conclusion of the argument above?

A   The exercise of free will is a relatively rare occurrence.

B   Most people never exercise free will.

C   The exercise of free will requires at least a certain degree of indeterminacy.

D   The universe is mostly deterministic.

E   Undetermined actions can be life-changing.

7. There is ample scientific evidence that, compared to teetotalers, people who drink red wine in moderate amounts (up to two glasses a day) enjoy better health and a prolonged life expectancy. Therefore, drinking red wine in moderate amounts is good for your health.

Which of the following is the best statement of the flaw in the above argument?

A   Many people do not drink any alcohol at all.

B   People tend to underreport how much alcohol they drink.

C   The kind of people who drink red wine in moderate amounts may have other protective factors in their diets or lifestyles.

D   Most of the scientific evidence in question was gathered by the wine industry.

E   Drinking red wine in excessive amounts is bad for your health.

8. The essence of the manic defence is to prevent feelings of helplessness and despair from entering into the conscious mind by occupying it with opposite feelings of euphoria, purposeful activity, and omnipotent control. That is why people feel driven not only to mark but also to celebrate such depressing milestones as entering the workforce (graduation), getting ever older (birthdays, New Year), and even, more recently, death and dying (Halloween). The manic defence may also take on more subtle forms, such as creating a commotion over something trivial; filling every 'spare moment' with reading, study, or on the phone to a friend; spending several months preparing for Christmas or some civic or sporting event; seeking out status or celebrity so as to be a 'somebody' rather than a 'nobody'; entering into baseless friendships and relationships; even, sometimes, getting married and having children.

Which of the following, if true, would most strengthen the above argument?

A Everyone uses the manic defence to varying degrees.

B The manic defence explains why airport shops are so profitable.

C The manic defence is an entirely subconscious process.

D The manic defence is especially prevalent in Occidental and Occidentalised societies.

E Some theories about human behaviour are difficult to falsify (prove to be false).

9. Mr Smith has to renew the white lines on a 2km stretch of road.

Each edge of the road is marked with a solid line and there is a dashed line in the centre. Drivers are warned of approaching bends by two curved arrows. Mr Smith will have to paint eight curved arrows.

The manufacturers have printed the following guidance on each 5L drum of paint:

– Solid lines: 5m per litre

– Dashed lines: 20m per litre

– Curved arrows: 3 litres each

How many drums of paint will Mr Smith require?

A 800

B 164

C 185

D 780

E 924

10. The chart shows the turnover of small businesses in North Oxford, according to a recent survey. The number of businesses per group is shown in parentheses.

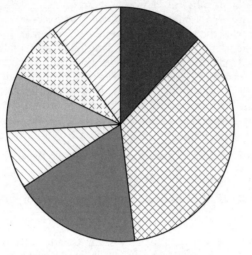

■ < £100K (6)   ⊠ £100K-250K (18)   ■ £250K-500K (9)   ◇ £500K-1M (4)

▦ £1M-3M (4)   ◌ £3M-10M (4)   ▨ > £10M (5)

What percentage of organisations has a turnover of £1M or less?

A   64%

B   68%

C   70%

D   74%

E   78%

11. The diagram shows the dimensions of an office and entry lobby. Both are to be carpeted. Each must have a single piece of carpet with no joins, although two separate pieces for the two rooms can be used.

Offcut pieces of carpet cost £10 per square metre.

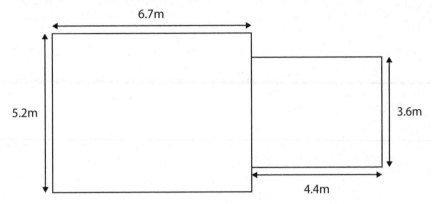

Which of the following offcut pieces will be suited to the job **and** work out cheapest?

A   8.6 x 5.5m

B   6.7 x 8.8m

C   6.7 x 9.6m

D   5.2 x 10.3m

E   5.2 x 11.1m

12. The increase in illegal human trafficking is one of the darker sides of globalisation. Legalising prostitution reduces illegal human trafficking. Despite raising overall demand for prostitution, customers will favour legal over trafficked prostitutes, thus reducing the demand for the latter. This is one example of how domestic policies crafted at the country level can still exert an impact on aspects of globalisation.

Which of the following is an underlying assumption of the argument above?

A   Legalising prostitution reduces illegal human trafficking.

B   The increase in the overall demand for prostitution does not lead to an overall increase in human trafficking.

C   Globalisation had led to an increase in illegal human trafficking.

D   The legalisation of prostitution leads customers to favour legal over trafficked prostitutes.

E   Globalisation can be shaped and controlled at the country level.

13. The longer one is alive, the more one 'accumulates' life. In contrast, death cannot be accumulated—it is not, as Nagel puts it, 'an evil of which Shakespeare has so far received a larger portion than Proust'. Most people would not consider the temporary suspension of life as an evil, nor would they regard the long period of time before they were born as an evil. Therefore, if death is an evil, this is not because it involves a period of non-existence, but because it deprives us of life.

Which of the following, if true, would most strengthen the above argument?

A   Unless something actually causes us displeasure, it cannot be an evil.

B   In the case of death, there is no longer a subject to suffer evil. Once a person has died, he no longer exists, and if he no longer exists, he cannot suffer evil.

C   People have no reason to regard the period of time after they are dead any differently to the period of time before they are born.

D   The good or evil that befalls a person depends on his history and possibilities rather than on his momentary state, which means that a person can suffer evil even if he is not here to experience it.

E   The time after a person's death is time in which he could have continued to enjoy the good of living.

14. A survey of voting intentions is carried out amongst various population groups in Oxfordshire.

	Group A	Group B	Group C	Group D	Total
Conservative	40	62	54	101	257
Labour	25	44	50	10	129
Lib Dem	9	28	55	24	115
Other	2	0	56	11	69
Total	76	134	215	145	570

One of the individual entries is incorrect, although marginal totals are correct.

Which is it?

A   24

B   10

C   55

D   25

E   40

15. 32 teams participate in a football tournament.

The teams are divided into four groups of eight teams. Within each group, each team plays each other team once. The top two teams in each group play in quarter-finals, with the winning team progressing to semi-finals, and the winning team of the semi-finals progressing to the final.

How many matches are there in total?

A   81

B   65

C   119

D   126

E   127

16. The triangle below may be cut into four identical pieces.

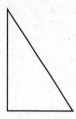

Which of the following pieces can be used four times (flips and rotations are allowed) to make up the triangle?

A

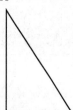

B

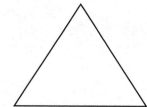

C

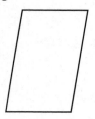

D

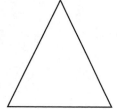

E

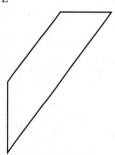

17. *Wuthering Heights* is the best book ever written in the English language. Each year for the past ten years, it has received more votes than any other book in our survey of British readers.

Which of the following is the best statement of the flaw in the above argument?

A   It assumes that a result is more valid if it is repeated over time.

B   It assumes that the British public have read every single book ever published in the English language.

C   It assumes that the sample surveyed was representative of the British public.

D   It assumes that popularity is the only measure of the quality of a book.

E   It assumes that the British public knows best.

18. The effectiveness of antidepressants has been greatly exaggerated. An influential paper combined 35 studies submitted to the Food and Drugs Administration (FDA) before the licensing of four antidepressants. The authors of the study found that, while the antidepressants performed better than a placebo, the effect size was very small for all but very severe cases of depression. _____, the authors attributed this increased effect size in very severe cases of depression not to an increase in the effect of the antidepressants, but to a decrease in the placebo effect.

Which of the following phrases, inserted in the blank space, most logically completes the above argument?

A   In conclusion,

B   However,

C   Therefore,

D   Similarly,

E   Moreover,

19. Alice is gifted in the arts. She has very good taste.

Which one of the following, if true, would most weaken the above argument?

A   Some people who are gifted in the arts are highly creative.

B   People who are gifted in the arts need not necessarily have good taste.

C   Many people who have good taste are not gifted in the arts.

D   Having good taste and being gifted in the arts are highly correlated.

E   Artists need to have inspiration and ability, as well as good taste.

20. The clock on Tom Tower is broken. It does tell the correct time, but only once every hour on the hour. The minute hand travels four times as fast down to 6 as it does back up to 12.

What is the correct time when the clock on Tom Tower shows half past one?

A   8 minutes past one

B   10 minutes past one.

C   11 minutes past one

D   12 minutes past one.

E   15 minutes past one.

21. Three years ago, Tom and Mary bought a house for £400,000. The house has gone up by 10% each year.

How much is the house now worth?

A   £430,000

B   £445,400

C   £520,000

D   £532,400

E   £560,000

22. In a seminar room, there are four tables, each identical to the one below.

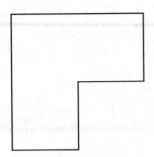

Which of the following arrangements is it **not** possible to make by putting the tables together?

A

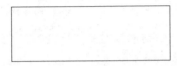

B

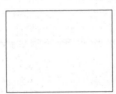

C

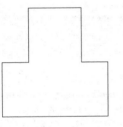

D

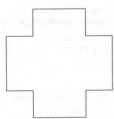

E

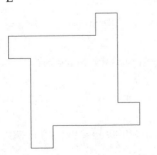

23. Before going grocery shopping, Amanda makes a list of exceptional items that she needs to buy. When she goes to the supermarket, she walks down every aisle, picking up her regular items such as milk and bread and trying as best as possible to remember to pick up the exceptional items as well. When she has been through every aisle, she looks at her list to check that she has not forgotten anything.

Which one the following uses the same method as that above?

A   Throughout the tax year, Adam compiles a list of all his income and expenditure in a notebook. When it comes to filing his taxes, he transfers all the information in his notebook onto his tax return.

B   Throughout the tax year, Adam compiles a list of all his income and expenditure in a notebook. When it comes to filing his taxes, he lists his income and expenditure from memory, and then checks his notebook to make sure that everything has been included.

C   Throughout the tax year, Adam compiles a list of exceptional income and expenditure in a notebook. When it comes to filing his taxes, he lists his regular income and expenditure from memory. He then refers to his notebook and lists any exceptional income and expenditure.

D   Throughout the tax year, Adam compiles a list of exceptional income and expenditure in a notebook. When it comes to filing his taxes, he lists his regular income and expenditure, and as much of his exceptional income and expenditure as he can recall. He does not refer back to his notebook.

E   Throughout the tax year, Adam compiles a list of exceptional income and expenditure in a notebook. When it comes to filing his taxes, he lists his regular income and expenditure, and as much of his exceptional income and expenditure as he can recall. He then checks his notebook to make sure that everything has been included.

24. The underlying nature of reality is unknowable. For even if sense experience is objective, which it is not, the underlying nature of reality cannot be observed through sense experience. Thus, the best that can be hoped for is not knowledge, but true belief.

Which of the following is an underlying assumption of the argument above?

A   Sense experience is not objective.

B   The underlying nature of reality cannot be observed through sense experience.

C   Knowledge of the underlying nature of reality can only be gained through sense experience.

D   Knowledge of the underlying nature of reality cannot be gained through sense experience.

E   True belief is equivalent to knowledge.

25. The UK government aims to improve access to university education for young people from disadvantaged backgrounds. However, whereas it used to provide students with maintenance grants that did not require repayment, it now provides the students with loans that they must gradually repay once they graduate and enter paid employment. The available evidence is that the prospect of debt is more likely to put off students from poorer families from going to university.

Which of the following is a conclusion that can be drawn from the above argument?

A   The loan system is fairer to the UK taxpayer.

B   The government's action goes against its aim.

C   The government's action supports its aim.

D   The maintenance grants had become unaffordable.

E   Students from poorer families are less ambitious.

26. Annual sales of a once fashionable toy fell by 40% in 2013 and by 75% in 2014.

By how much must sales increase in 2015 if they are to match original sales?

A   85%

B   667%

C   115%

D   150%

E   500%

27. The table shows government debt and population levels for Eurozone countries in 2012.

Country	Government Debt 2012 (€ millions)	Population 2012	Percent
Ireland	192,461	4,495,351	1.4%
Belgium	375,389	11,041,266	3.3%
Italy	1,988, 658	60,850,782	18.3%
France	1,833,810	65,397,912	19.6%
Austria	227,431	8,443,018	2.5%
Greece	303,918	11,290,785	3.4%
Germany	2,166,278	81,843,809	24.6%
Netherlands	427,515	16,730,348	5.0%
Portugal	204,485	10,541,840	3.2%
Spain	883,873	46,196,277	13.9%
Finland	103,131	5,401,267	1.6%
Cyprus	15,350	862,011	0.3%
Luxembourg	9,232	524,853	0.2%
Malta	4,871	420,085	0.1%
Slovenia	19,189	2,055,496	0.6%
Slovakia	37,245	5,404,322	1.6%
Estonia	1,724	1,339,662	0.4%
Total/Average	8,794,559	332,839,084	100.0%

What is the minimum number of countries needed to make up at least 50% of the Eurozone population?

A   2

B   3

C   4

D   5

E   6

28. The table shows the share price in pence for *** Inc. from May 1 to May 15.

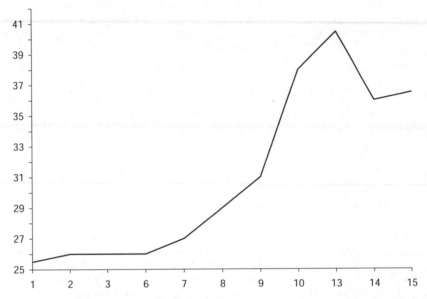

- *** Inc. has 250,000,000 shares in issue.
- The offer price to buy shares is 1p above the share price.
- The bid price to sell shares is 1p below the share price.
- Upon buying, a tax of 0.5% of the total value of the transaction (not including the transaction fee) must be paid.
- The transaction fee for buying and selling is £20.
- The opening price on a particular day is the closing price of the previous trading day. For example, the opening price on the 2nd of May is 26p, which is also the closing price on the 1st of May.
- Shares are not traded on Saturdays, Sundays, and Bank Holidays.
- Capital gains tax is charged at a flat rate of 20% on all profit.

What is the value of the company based on the closing price on 13th May?

A   £90m

B   £80m

C   £70m

D   £100m

E   £101m

29. The acts that people call altruistic are in fact selfish. For example, they may be underpinned by the expectation of honour or reciprocation or the greater likelihood of a place in heaven. At the very least, altruistic acts relieve unpleasant feelings such as the guilt or shame of not having acted, and lead to pleasant feelings of pride and satisfaction.

    Which of the following is the best statement of the flaw in the above argument?

    A   The acts that people call altruistic are variously self-motivated.

    B   The acts that people call altruistic involve at least an element of self-interest.

    C   The acts that people call altruistic involve an inevitable element of self-interest.

    D   The fact that altruistic acts involve an inevitable element of self-interest need not mean that they are selfish.

    E   People may have mixed motives.

30. Social phobia has many features in common with shyness, and distinguishing between the two can be a cause for debate and controversy. Some critics have gone so far as to suggest that 'social phobia' is nothing more than a convenient label used to pass off a personality trait as a mental disorder and to legitimise its medical 'treatment'. _____ it can be argued that social phobia differs from shyness in that it starts at a later age and is more severe and debilitating.

    Which of the following phrases, inserted in the blank space, most logically completes the above argument?

    A   Indeed,

    B   Moreover,

    C   According to them,

    D   However,

    E   In contrast,

31. The existence of laws implies the existence of lawgivers. There are laws in nature. Therefore, there must be a cosmic lawgiver.

Which of the following most closely parallels the reasoning in the above argument?

A   A feather is light. What is light cannot be dark. Therefore, a feather cannot be dark.

B   There is no smoke without a fire. There is smoke. Therefore, there is a fire.

C   Unless I get at least three As, I will not become a doctor. I didn't get at least three A's. Therefore, I will not become a doctor.

D   No handymen are bakers. No bakers are fishermen. Therefore, no handymen are fishermen.

E   If I drop an egg it breaks. This egg is broken. Therefore, I must have dropped it.

32. A particular textbook normally costs £25.

However, the publisher offers course organisers certain levels of discounts if they buy the book in bulk, as follows:

Number of books purchased	Discount
10–25	20%
26–39	25%
40–100	40%
101+	50%

Dr Pideritt uses the textbook as a set text for his course. This year, 36 students will require the textbook.

How much would Dr Pideritt save if he bought 40 copies rather than 36?

A   £20

B   £45

C   £90

D   £60

E   £75

33. A teacher noticed that there were fewer than 100 pupils in the playground. When she counted them by 2s, there was one pupil left over. She then counted them by 3s, 4s, 5s, and 6s, and found that, in each case, there was one pupil left over.

How many pupils were there in the playground?

A 57

B 61

C 69

D 87

E 93

34. The chart shows the average amount of rainfall per month in millimetres in a particular wine region.

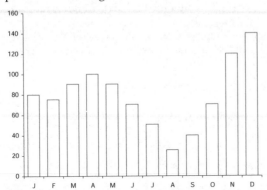

Which one of the following graphs could show the monthly change in average rainfall?

A

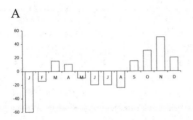

B

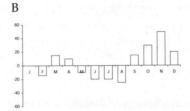

C

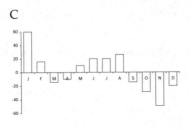

D

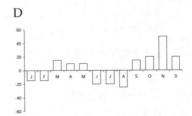

E

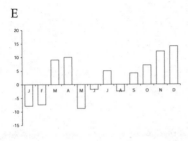

35. The rate of growth of grass dramatically reduces during the winter months, and so most people do not mow their lawns in the winter. However, mowing the lawn every three or four weeks in winter (at a relatively high level) can really lift a winterised garden, leaving the garden's centrepiece looking even and beautifully striped. Also, when spring arrives, the grass will be thicker and more vigorous. Therefore, people should be encouraged to mow their lawn throughout the winter.

Which one of the following, if true, would most strengthen the above argument?

A   Grass stops growing when the air temperature falls below about 5°C.

B   Most people need more exercise, particularly during the winter months.

C   Mowing the lawn in winter helps to remove leaf litter and debris.

D   Walking over a frosted lawn damages the grass.

E   In winter, factors such as reduced daylight hours, cold temperatures, and water logging limit opportunities to mow the lawn.

36. The values of equality, fairness, and political correctness that have come to pervade almost every aspect of public life in Britain are completely alien to traditional societies and completely alien even to the Britain of not so long ago, which, among others, governed the largest empire that history records. Other examples of values that are far from timeless and universal include those surrounding risk ('health and safety'), ideal body image, premarital and homosexual sexual relations, single parenting, and the rearing of children.

Which of the following summarises the conclusion of the argument above?

A   Some of the values that have come to pervade public life in Britain are not timeless and universal.

B   The values held by a society can change very fast.

C   Values have progressed since the decline of the British Empire.

D   Values are groundless.

E   Values are constantly changing.

37. Mr and Mrs Smith were at the garden centre when Mrs Smith, who was heavily pregnant, began to experience her first contractions. Mr Smith maintained that it would be quicker to drive Mrs Smith to the hospital than to call for an ambulance. By the time they got into the car, Mrs Smith was in great distress. She pleaded with Mr Smith to drive faster, but he refused to do so on the grounds that it is prohibited to exceed the legal speed limit.

Which of the following most closely parallels the reasoning in the above argument?

A   Tom and Harry were stuck in a traffic jam on the motorway. Harry wanted to get home to watch the live football, so he asked Tom to drive on the hard shoulder. However, Tom refused to do so on the grounds that it is prohibited to drive on a hard shoulder.

B   Tom and Harry were stuck in a traffic jam on the motorway. Harry had a bad case of diarrhoea, so he asked Tom to drive on the hard shoulder. Tom felt sorry for Harry and agreed to drive on the hard shoulder.

C   I try as much as possible to avoid hurting animals on the grounds that it is cruel and wrong. That's why I'm a vegetarian.

D   Nowadays, domesticated meat animals are slaughtered in such a way that they do not suffer any pain. So, although I believe that it is wrong to hurt animals, I still do eat meat.

E   My house is infested with rats. But it is wrong to hurt animals, so I can't do anything about it.

38. John is older than Sarah and Sarah is younger than Freddy.

Freddy is older than John, but younger than Mary.

Mary is:

A   The youngest

B   Younger than Sarah

C   Older than John, but younger than Freddy

D   Younger than Sarah and Freddy

E   The oldest

39. The cost of publishing a 200-page book is £4,000. 40% of this goes on typesetting, 50% on printing, and 10% on cover design. For a 300-page book, the cost of typesetting increases by 25% and the cost of printing by 15%. The cost of cover design stays the same.

How much does it cost to publish a 300-page book?

A   £4,500

B   £4,600

C   £4,700

D   £4,800

E   £4,900

40. Oliver received a novelty wine rack for Christmas. He got bored half way through Christmas lunch and started counting the triangles in the wine rack.

What is the highest number of triangles he could have counted?

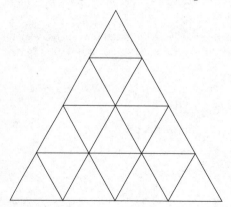

A   17

B   23

C   27

D   25

E   31

41. For many people living in our society, life can seem both suffocating and far removed, lonely even and especially among the multitudes, and not only meaningless but absurd. By encoding their distress in terms of depression or another mental disorder, our society may be subtly implying that the problem lies not with itself but with them, fragile and failing individuals that they are. Of course, many people prefer to buy into this reductive, physicalist explanation than to confront their existential angst. But thinking of unhappiness in terms of an illness or chemical imbalance in the brain can be counterproductive, as it can prevent people from identifying and addressing the important psychological or life problems that are at the root of their distress.

Which of the following, if true, would most strengthen the above argument?

A   There is strong evidence that mental disorders such as depression result from a chemical imbalance in the brain.

B   There is strong evidence that antidepressants are very effective.

C   Depression is very rarely witnessed in traditional or historical societies.

D   The average consultation with a doctor is about eight minutes long.

E   Pharmaceutical companies fund much of the research into mental health.

42. The social drinking of wine, during or after a meal, and in full cognizance of its delicate taste and evocative aura, seldom leads to drunkenness, and yet more seldom to loutish behaviour. The drink problem that we witness in British cities stems from our inability to pay Bacchus [an ancient god of wine] his due. Thanks to cultural impoverishment, young people no longer have a repertoire of songs, poems, arguments, or ideas with which to entertain one another in their cups. They drink to fill the moral vacuum generated by their culture, and while we are familiar with the adverse effect of drink on an empty stomach, we are now witnessing the far worse effect of drink on an empty mind.

Which of the following is an underlying assumption of the argument above?

A   The drink problem in British cities is worse than it used to be.

B   There is no drink problem in rural Britain.

C   Older people are not affected by cultural impoverishment.

D   Culture can provide us with a moral framework.

E   Wine ought to be drunk with respect and reverence.

43. All humans are mortal. Greeks are humans. Therefore Greeks are mortal.

Which of the following most closely parallels the reasoning in the above argument?

A   No reptiles have fur. All snakes are reptiles. Therefore no snakes have fur.

B   All rabbits have fur. Some pets are rabbits. Therefore some pets have fur.

C   Some cats have no tails. All cats are mammals. Therefore some mammals have no tails.

D   All mortals die. All men are mortals. Therefore all men die.

E   All men are mortal. All Greeks are men. Therefore some Greeks are mortal.

44. Two private tutors, Mr Sanders and Mrs Patel, charge the same hourly rate of £60 per hour. However, if the student books more than four hours, Mr Sanders reduces his rate to £50 per hour for the entirety of the booking, while Mrs Patel offers an extra 40 minutes per 4 hours booked.

Assuming that Mr Sanders and Mrs Patel are equally good tutors, how much would John save if he wanted 14 hours of tuition and booked Mr Sanders instead of Mrs Patel?

A   £10

B   £20

C   £35

D   £50

E   £80

45. Various shapes may be made by overlapping two transparent triangles, for example, as in this case, an equilateral triangle.

Which one of the following shapes cannot be made by overlapping the two transparent triangles?

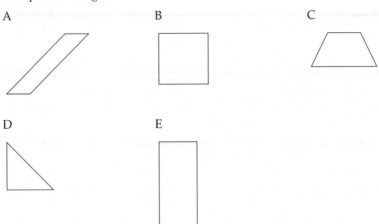

A

B

C

D

E

46. According to some educational experts, the term 'dyslexia' should be ditched because it is unscientific and lacks educational value. The experts argue that putting young people who are struggling to read through diagnostic tests is a waste of resources, because the label lacks meaning. The focus should be on helping children to read, rather than finding a label for their difficulty. Parents are being woefully misled about the value of a dyslexia diagnosis, which is often undermining and distressing to children.

Which of the following best expresses the main conclusion of the argument above?

A   The focus should be on helping children to read, rather than finding a label for their difficulty.

B   The term 'dyslexia' should be ditched.

C   The term 'dyslexia' is unscientific and lacks educational value.

D   Putting young people who are struggling to read through diagnostic tests is a waste of resources.

E   Parents are being misled about the value of a dyslexia diagnosis.

47. If two patients need a heart transplant to survive, and there is only one heart available, the heart should go to the person who will, on the balance of probabilities, make the greatest contribution to society.

Which one of the following is **least** illustrative of the principle underlying the above argument?

A   In general, it is wrong to torture people. But in some cases, a criminal or prisoner of war could be tortured if doing so would provide intelligence information that could make the majority of people safer.

B   In the early 1990s, some people in South Africa argued that apartheid [a system of racial segregation] should be maintained on the grounds that allowing the black majority to run the government—although the right thing to do in principle—could lead to civil wars, economic decline, famine, and unrest.

C   The principle to 'always tell the truth' promotes the general good, and so should always be followed—even if in a particular situation lying would produce the best consequences.

D   Although potentially harmful, cannabis should be legalised, regulated, and taxed, just like alcohol or tobacco. This would increase tax revenues, reduce policing and legal costs, and end the persecution of harmless people.

E   The bombing of Hiroshima and Nagasaki by the United States was morally justified. Yes, it did kill thousands of Japanese—but it also put an end to the war between the United States and Japan before other countries could get involved. Without the bombing, it is likely that many more innocent people would have died.

48. No dogs are birds. Some mammals are dogs. Therefore some mammals are not birds.

Which of the following most closely parallels the reasoning in the above argument?

A   No birds are mammals. Some animals are birds. Therefore some animals are not mammals.

B   No reptiles have fur. All snakes are reptiles. Therefore no snakes have fur.

C   All birds are animals. All parrots are birds. Therefore all parrots are animals.

D   No birds are foxes. All parrots are birds. Therefore no parrots are foxes.

E   No dogs are birds. Some birds are pets. Therefore some pets are not dogs.

49. 250 people apply for tax advice. Of these, 180 are self-employed and 50 are in online retailing. Only 40 people are neither self-employed nor in online retailing.

How many people are both self-employed and in online retailing?

A   10

B   15

C   20

D   30

E   35

50. Some of the squares on a 4x4 board are marked with certain symbols, which may or may not be covered up by a circular counter. At one stage in the game, the board looks like this (all the circles represent counters which cover up the square that they occupy).

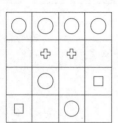

Which of the following represents a possible layout of the board (not necessarily viewed in the same direction as above)?

A

B

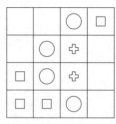

C

D

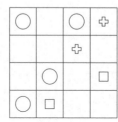

E

Paper 3

1. For Aristotle, it is by understanding the distinctive function of a thing that one can understand its essence. For example, one cannot understand what it is to be a gardener unless one can understand that the distinctive function of a gardener is 'to tend to a garden with a certain degree of skill'. Whereas human beings need nourishment like plants and have sentience like animals, their distinctive function, says Aristotle, is their unique capacity to reason. Thus, the Supreme Good, or Happiness, for human beings is to lead a life that enables them to exercise and to develop their reason, and that is in accordance with rational principles. In contrast to amusement or pleasure, which can be enjoyed even by animals, happiness is not a state but an activity, and it is profound and enduring.

   Which of the following is an underlying assumption of the argument above?

   A   The essence of a gardener is to garden with skill.

   B   Human beings should not pursue amusement or pleasure.

   C   The capacity to reason is unique to human beings.

   D   The Supreme Good for a thing is for it to exercise its distinctive function.

   E   The Supreme Good for human beings is to exercise and develop their reason.

2. Spontaneous human combustion (SHC) is a term encompassing the rare reported cases of the burning of a living human body without an apparent external source of ignition. People who believe in SHC have come up with all sorts of theories to explain the phenomenon, ranging from a 'visitation from God' to the pyrotron theory, which stipulates the existence of a subatomic particle that is able to ignite a combustible source. These and other fanciful theories can be dismissed owing to two quite mundane observations. First, there is always a period of at least a few hours between the time a victim is last seen alive and the time that he or she is found immolated. Second, there is always a nearby source of ignition. Cases of apparent SHC are simply those rare cases where a natural death in isolation has been followed by a slow combustion from some nearby source of ignition.

   Which of the following is an underlying assumption of the argument above?

   A   SHC does not exist.

   B   Reported cases of the phenomenon termed SHC are rare.

   C   Reported cases of the phenomenon termed SHC need to be accurately documented.

   D   Where there are competing explanations for an unexplained phenomenon, the more commonly held one ought to prevail.

   E   Where there are competing explanations for an unexplained phenomenon, the more simple or ordinary one ought to prevail.

3. Young motorists have been thrown a lifeline in the battle against soaring motor insurance costs after one of Britain's biggest insurers launched a new Smartbox that will monitor how they drive, and reward safe motoring with cheaper premiums. This 'pay how you drive' scheme should encourage young motorists to drive more carefully, and thereby lead to an overall fall in their insurance premiums. However, whereas good driving will be rewarded, bad driving will be penalised with higher premiums. Young motorists who have been driving recklessly will be in for an increased premium, of up to 15 per cent, whereas good driving will be rewarded with discounts of up to 11 per cent. So, whereas the scheme will encourage young drivers to drive more carefully, it will not lead to an overall fall in their insurance premiums.

   Which of the following, if true, would most weaken the above argument?

   A   Young motorists who drive recklessly are more likely to forfeit their driving license, and so no longer require insurance.

   B   Under the scheme, young motorists who speed will receive an email warning them that they have been driving badly.

   C   An 11 per cent discount is too small to alter driving habits.

   D   The vast majority of young motorists under the scheme will drive responsibly.

   E   Unlike traditional insurance, which remains at a fixed quoted price for a whole year, the pay-how-you-drive-system will be recalculated every 90 days.

4. In a certain wine-producing region, the number of vines planted out in a vineyard is directly proportional to its area.

   A 100m by 40m vineyard counts 1,440 vines.

   How many vines are there in a 300m x 80m vineyard?

   A   6,400

   B   6,820

   C   7,600

   D   8,640

   E   8,660

5. In order to destroy a ballistic missile, a fighter jet must be almost level with it.

   An RAF jet travelling at 720km/h is chasing a ballistic missile travelling at 500km/h over the Arctic Ocean. The jet and the missile are 110km apart.

   How long will it take the jet to catch up with the missile?

   A   15 minutes

   B   30 minutes

   C   60 minutes

   D   130 minutes

   E   220 minutes

6. Eloise is on a skiing holiday. One morning, she takes a ski lift to the top of a slope and then skis all the way back to the bottom of the ski lift. The ski lift is parallel to the ski run, such that they both cover exactly the same distance.

   The ski lift travels at a constant speed of 5km/hr. Eloise skis down the slope at an average speed of 20km/hr.

   The round trip takes her 30 minutes.

   How long is the ski run?

   A   2.0km

   B   2.4km

   C   3.2 km

   D   3.6km

   E   4.0km

7. While personality disorders may lead to distress and impairment, they may also lead to extraordinary achievement. In 2005, Board and Fritzon found that, compared to mentally disordered criminal offenders at the high security Broadmoor Hospital, high-level executives were more likely to have one of three personality disorders: histrionic personality disorder, narcissistic personality disorder, and anankastic personality disorder. Thus, it is possible to envisage that people may benefit from strongly ingrained and potentially maladaptive traits. In their study, Board and Fritzon described the executives with a personality disorder as 'successful psychopaths' and the criminal offenders as 'unsuccessful psychopaths', and it may be that highly successful and disturbed psychopaths have more in common than first meets the eye. As William James put it more than a hundred years ago, 'When a superior intellect and a psychopathic temperament coalesce … in the same individual, we have the best possible condition for the kind of effective genius that gets into the biographical dictionaries.'

Which of the following best expresses the main conclusion of the argument above?

A All psychopaths have a lot in common.

B Most highly successful people are psychopaths.

C High-level executives are more likely to have a personality disorder than mentally disordered criminal offenders at Broadmoor Hospital.

D People may benefit from strongly ingrained and potentially maladaptive traits.

E The difference between a successful psychopath and an unsuccessful psychopath is mostly one of intelligence.

8. Genes for debilitating disorders such as bipolar disorder usually pass out of the population over time because affected people have fewer children. The fact that this has not happened for bipolar disorder suggests that the responsible genes are being maintained despite their debilitating effects on a significant proportion of the population, and thus that they are conferring an important adaptive or evolutionary advantage that promotes their survival in the population.

Which of the following, if true, would most strengthen the above argument?

A Bipolar disorder is not a genetic disorder.

B Despite their debilitating illness, people with bipolar disorder have more children.

C Bipolar disorder is more common in higher socioeconomic groups.

D Bipolar disorder is more common in lower socioeconomic groups.

E Ernest Hemingway, who won the Nobel Prize in literature, suffered from bipolar disorder.

9. When Nathan moved to London, he could either have bought a property or rented one. Although buying a place would have been a better investment, he could not afford the sort of deposit required for a London property. So he had no choice but to rent. In the end, he got together with some friends and rented a room in a shared flat.

   Which one of the following most closely parallels the kind of reasoning used in the passage above?

   A You can buy this book in a bookshop or online. If you buy it online it will be cheaper, but you will have to wait longer to start reading it.

   B There are two dentists working at the practice. The man is very competent and professional, while the woman is rude and questionable. Make sure to ask for the man.

   C We could go out for dinner or stay at home and cook a meal. I've just remembered: there are no ingredients at home. That leaves us no option but to go out for dinner.

   D We could go out for dinner or stay at home and cook a meal. I know you would rather stay at home and save money, but I'm quite tired, so let's go out and I'll invite you.

   E The trail is used by both hikers and bikers. If you're a hiker, you might as well assume that the bikers have the right-of-way, because that's the way most bikers behave.

10. Eloise is on a skiing holiday. One morning, she takes a ski lift and gets into chair number 15.

    Exactly half way to the top of the slope, she passes chair number 92 on its way down.

    How many chairs are there on the ski lift?

    You can assume that the chairs are evenly spaced and sequentially numbered from number 1.

    A 76

    B 100

    C 152

    D 154

    E 162

11. A taxi driver charges a fixed fare plus an amount that varies according to the time of day. Between 6pm and 10pm, that variable amount doubles, and between 10pm and 6am it quadruples.

Which one of the following price scales would fit his pricing scheme?

A   £3.50, £5.00, £7.50

B   £5.00, £7.00, £9.00

C   £5.00, £7.00, £11.00

D   £4.50, £7.00, £12.00

E   £4.00, £6.00, £9.50

12. In a primary school classroom, there are six tables, each identical to the one below.

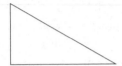

Which of the following arrangements is it not possible to make by putting the tables together?

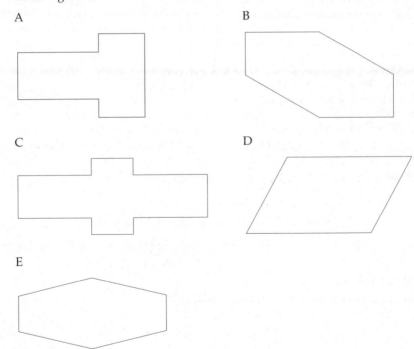

A

B

C

D

E

13. Even if God exists, and even if He had an intelligent purpose in creating humankind, we do not know what this predetermined purpose might be and, whatever it might be, we would rather be able to do without it. Unless we can be free to become the authors of our own purpose or purposes, our lives may have, at worse, no purpose at all, and, at best, only some unfathomable and potentially trivial purpose that is not of our choosing.

Which of the following is an underlying assumption of the argument above?

A   Having the freedom to choose our own purpose is necessarily better than having a predetermined purpose, whatever it might be.

B   God does not exist.

C   For something to have a purpose, it must necessarily have been created with that purpose in mind.

D   Something that was created with a purpose in mind must necessarily have the same purpose for which it was created.

E   We should strive to create our own purpose or purposes.

14. The majority of medical conditions are defined by their cause ('aetiology') or by the damage to the body that they result from ('pathology'), and so are relatively easy to define and recognise. If a person is suspected of having malaria, a blood sample can be taken and examined under a microscope for malarial parasites; and if a person is suspected of having had a cerebral infarction (or stroke), a brain scan can be taken to look for evidence of obstruction of an artery in the brain. In contrast, mental disorders are concepts that so far can only be defined by their supposed predominant symptoms. For example, if a person is suspected of having schizophrenia, there are no laboratory or physical tests that can objectively confirm the diagnosis. Instead, the psychiatrist must base his diagnosis solely on the symptoms manifested by the patient, without the help of any tests. If the symptoms tally with those by which schizophrenia is defined, then the psychiatrist is able to make a diagnosis of schizophrenia.

Which of the following conclusions is best supported by the above passage?

A   The definitions of mental disorders are circular.

B   Mental disorders are defined either by their aetiology or by their pathology.

C   Mental disorders are relatively easy to define and recognise.

D   Mental disorders are concepts that so far can only be defined by their supposed predominant symptoms.

E   The definition of schizophrenia is circular.

15. The table shows the driving distance between various hospitals in miles.

John Radcliffe				
2	Churchill			
29	31	Horton		
29	28	70	Royal Berkshire	
22	23	39	39	Stoke Mandeville

A doctor drives from the John Radcliffe to the Horton in the morning, and then from the Horton to the Churchill in the afternoon.

He receives mileage of 40p per mile for the first 40 miles driven in a day, and then just 30p per mile. How much mileage money is he owed?

A   £20

B   £22

C   £24

D   £18

E   £26

16. Chrissie is running a one-day course for 20 students.

She charges each student £200 to attend the course.

She must pay:

– £250 for advertising the course

– £1,400 to rent the venue for the course

– £150 to rent the laptop, projector, and screen

– £2 per student for coffee in the morning break

– £20 per student for lunch

– £4 per student for tea and cakes in the afternoon break

She must also print a 220-page hand-out for each student. The cost of printing is 20p per page plus £5 for binding (per hand-out).

How much profit does she make from running the course?

A   £150

B   £400

C   £700

D   £1,100

E   £1,680

17. The figure shows expected peak flow rates of air upon breathing out as hard as possible into a peak flow meter (essentially a tube).

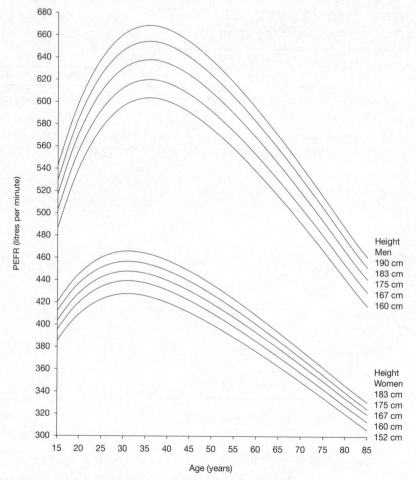

What **cannot** be said about expected peak flow rates in men compared to expected peak flow rates in women?

A   They are higher.

B   They peak later in life.

C   They have a larger range.

D   They do not overlap with those in women.

E   Once they have peaked, they fall off more rapidly with advancing age.

18. Don't be envious. Whenever you come across someone who is better or more successful than you are, you can react with either envy or emulation. Envy is the pain that you feel because others have good things; emulation is the pain that you feel because you yourself do not have them. This is a subtle but critical difference. Unlike envy, which is useless at best and self-defeating at worst, emulation is a good thing because it makes us take steps towards securing good things.

Which of the following best expresses the main conclusion of the argument above?

A   Emulation is a good thing.

B   Emulation is better than envy.

C   Don't be envious.

D   Whenever you come across someone who is better or more successful than you are, you can react with either envy or emulation.

E   Both envy and emulation involve pain.

19. All terriers are dogs. All terriers have strong hunting instincts. Therefore some dogs have strong hunting instincts.

Which of the following most closely parallels the reasoning in the above argument?

A   All butterflies are insects. All insects are invertebrates. Therefore all butterflies are invertebrates.

B   All butterflies are insects. Some butterflies are highly patterned. Therefore some insects are highly patterned.

C   All sculptors are artists. All sculptors are concerned with form. Therefore some artists are concerned with form.

D   All poets are artists. No artist is an island. Therefore no poet is an island.

E   All poets are artists. Some poets are not novelists. Therefore some artists are not novelists.

20. Flavius: Have you forgot me, sir?

Timon: Why dost ask that? I have forgot all men;

Then, if thou grant'st thou'rt a man, I have forgot thee.

Which of the following most closely parallels the reasoning in the above argument?

A   All psychiatrists are doctors. You are not a doctor. Therefore you are not a psychiatrist.

B   All doctors are accountable to a professional body. All psychiatrists are doctors. Therefore all psychiatrists are accountable to a professional body.

C   Some psychiatrists are psychotherapists. All psychotherapists are thoughtful. Therefore some psychiatrists are thoughtful.

D   All cowards inspire fear. Tim is a coward. Therefore Tim inspires fear.

E   I fear all cowards. You are a coward. Therefore I fear you.

21. A purse contains the same number of 1p coins, 5p coins, and 10p coins. The coins add up to £1.92.

How many of each type of coin does the purse contain?

A   9

B   10

C   11

D   12

E   13

22. Robert is driving to France from his home in Aylesbury, Buckinghamshire. He heads for the Ferry Port in Dover and boards a ferry.

The ferry has a deck area of 3,600m² for parking cars and coaches. Every car takes up 20m² and every coach takes up 80m².

The charge for a car is £50 and the charge for a coach is £200.

Each car carries an average of 2 passengers and each coach carries an average of 8 passengers. Each passenger spends an average of £15 on board the ferry.

Assuming the deck is full, how much money did the ferry operator take in?

A   £15,000

B   £14,400

C   £13,600

D   £11,000

E   £9,000

23. The diagram shows the outline of a window frame composed of identical pieces of wood, all of the same size and shape.

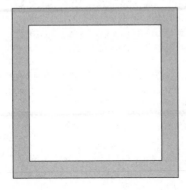

Which one of the following shapes could make up the window frame?

A

B

C

D

E

24. In modern societies such as the UK and the USA, people talk about depression more readily and more openly. As a result, they are more likely to interpret their distress in terms of depression, and less likely to fear stigma if they seek out a diagnosis of depression. At the same time, groups with vested interests such as pharmaceutical companies and mental health experts promote the notion of saccharine happiness as a natural, default state, and of human distress as a mental disorder. The concept of depression as a mental disorder may be useful for the more severe cases seen by hospital psychiatrists, but probably not for the majority of cases, which, for the most part, are mild and short-lived, and easily interpreted in terms of the human condition.

Which of the following is a statement of the main conclusion of the above argument?

A   People in modern societies are more likely to interpret their distress in terms of depression.

B   In modern societies, the concept of depression as a mental disorder has been overextended to include all manner of human suffering.

C   People in modern societies find it easier to think of their problems in terms of a mental disorder such as depression.

D   The concept of depression as a mental disorder is only useful for the more severe cases seen by hospital psychiatrists.

E   Thinking of unhappiness in terms of a mental disorder can be counterproductive because it can prevent people from identifying and addressing the important psychological or life problems that are at the root of their distress.

25. MBA degrees used to really help you stand out. Now that elite clique is more like a crowd. Decreasing salaries for MBA graduates combined with skyrocketing tuition costs mean that an MBA no longer guarantees a return on your investment. So instead of burdening yourself with $100,000 debt, you should try an internship or start your own business.

Which of the following, if true, would most strengthen the above argument?

A   In the last ten years, the number of MBAs awarded by US schools rose by 80%.

B   In the last ten years, average fees for an MBA rose by 65%.

C   Most networking now takes place over the internet and social media.

D   The new business landscape grants innovative, entrepreneurial, and ambitious people all sorts of new opportunities, without the degrees.

E   MBA professors may be smart theorists, but they are untested business people.

26. Every year, violent schizophrenics kill a number of people. The papers are full of such horrific cases. Schizophrenics should not be cared for in the community, but detained in perpetuity in secure units. This may deprive them of liberty, but what is liberty compared to life?

Which of the following is the best statement of the flaw in the above argument?

A   The papers over-report killings by schizophrenia sufferers.

B   Not all schizophrenia sufferers are violent or pose a risk to others.

C   Schizophrenia cannot be successfully treated.

D   The liberty of many can trump the life of a few.

E   People should be presumed innocent until proven guilty.

27. The Botanical Gardens in Middlemarch charge a day entry fee of £4.50 for adults and £3.00 for concessions, including children under the age of 16.

Also available is an annual pass, which costs £42 for adults and £28 for concessions.

Mr and Mrs Royston and their two children aged 12 and 10 plan to visit the garden 40 times this year.

How much would they save by buying annual passes?

A   £140

B   £260

C   £380

D   £460

E   £280

28. A winemaker buys £2,600 of grapes from a grower. The grower buys £2,200 of wine from the winemaker. The grower buys £600 of pesticide from a chemist. The winemaker buys £300 of cultured yeasts from the chemist. The chemist buys £600 of wine from the winemaker.

Which of the following will settle their accounts while minimising transaction costs?

A   The winemaker pays the grower £400 and the grower pays £600 to the chemist.

B   The winemaker pays the grower £100 and the grower pays the chemist £300.

C   The chemist pays £300 to the winemaker, and the grower pays £600 to the chemist.

D   The winemaker and the grower each pay the chemist £300.

E   The winemaker pays the chemist £100 and the grower pays the chemist £200.

29. The cost of renting a rowing boat for two hours is £18 plus £4 per person, up to a maximum of 6 people.

Which one of the following line graphs best illustrates the cost per person as more people club together to rent the boat?

A

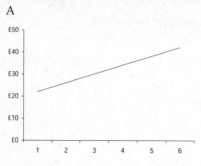

B

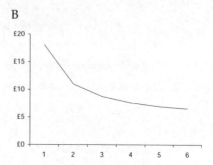

C

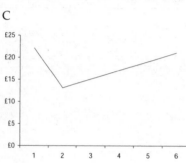

D

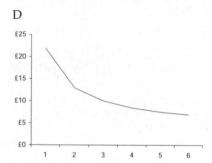

E

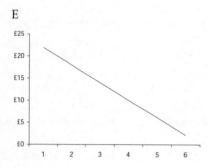

30. Non-insulin dependent diabetes mellitus (NIDDM) is a condition that is closely associated with obesity. A recent study by the pharmaceutical company that manufactures the most effective drug for the treatment of NIDDM found that prescription rates for the drug in people with a Body Mass Index (BMI) greater than 30 varied by more than fourfold from one English region to another. The study exposes the disastrous 'postcode lottery' of care within the health service, where the effectiveness of the treatment for a health condition depends upon where you live.

Which of the following is an underlying assumption of the argument above?

A   NIDDM is caused by obesity.

B   There are no regional variations in the numbers of people with a BMI greater than 30.

C   There are no regional variations in the prevalence of NIDDM in the population group under study.

D   The drug is much more effective than its alternatives.

E   The pharmaceutical company does not have a vested interest in publishing the study.

31. A study examined the careers of physicists who began publishing between 1950 and 1980 and continued to do so for at least 20 years. The researchers ranked the impact of the institutions that the physicists attended by counting the number of citations each institution's papers received within five years of publication. By tracking the affiliations of individual physicists and counting their citations in a similar way, they were able to work out whether moving from a low- to a high-ranking university improved a physicist's impact. In total, they analyzed 2,725 careers. They found that, though an average physicist moved once or twice during his career, moving from a low-rank university to an elite one did not increase his scientific impact. Going in the opposite direction, however, did have a small negative influence.

Which of the following is a conclusion than can be drawn from the above passage?

A   Physicists are not representative of academics as a whole.

B   Moving from a low-rank university to an elite one does not increase the scientific impact of the average physicist.

C   Moving from a low-rank university to an elite one does not increase the scientific impact of the average physicist; however, going in the opposite direction does have a small negative influence.

D   As far as physics is concerned, elite universities do not add value to output.

E   Authorities should not concentrate physics research into fewer, more elite institutions.

32. The City Council has built exercise stations in the arboretum [tree park] in the hope of attracting more visitors. Current users of the arboretum see it as a place of rest and contemplation, a sanctuary from the hustle and bustle of city living. They are strongly opposed to the exercise stations, and have petitioned the Council to have them removed. If the Council had carried out a proper public consultation, it would not have wasted public money on these exercise stations, money which would have been better spent on upgrading existing facilities for current users of the arboretum.

Which of the following is the best statement of the flaw in the above argument?

A   The Council cannot be sure that the exercise stations will attract new visitors.

B   Current visitors will continue to come in spite of the exercise stations.

C   The exercise stations will almost certainly attract some new visitors.

D   Money ought to be spent on actual rather than potential visitors.

E   Though unpopular with current visitors, the exercise stations may yet attract more visitors overall.

33. At the end of the season, Tom is top-dressing his lawn with a mixture of loam and sand. He has 500kg of top-dressing consisting of 70% loam and 30% sand. However, he would like the mixture to consist of 50% sand so as to improve drainage over the wet winter months.

How much sand does he have to add to the mixture?

A   150kg

B   200kg

C   250kg

D   100kg

E   300kg

34. A painter has to redecorate a room that is 9.5 metres long, 4.8 metres wide, and 3.2 metres high.

One of the long walls is not to be painted, but to be covered in wallpaper. The long wall has neither doors nor windows.

One roll of wallpaper is 60cm wide and 4m long.

Which mathematical formula represents the number of rolls of wallpaper that the painter will need?

A (9.5 x 4.8) x (60 x 4)

B (9.5 x 3.2)/(60 x 4)

C (9.5 x 4.8)/(0.6 x 4)

D (9.5 x 3.2) x (0.6 x 4)

E (9.5 x 3.2)/(0.6 x 4)

35. The fuel consumption of my hatchback is summarised in the table.

Speed (mph)	Consumption (l/100m)
30	10
50	12
70	15

Every day, I use the car to drive to and from work. The journey to work (one way) involves 5 miles on urban roads at 30mph, 20 miles on country roads at 50mph, and 30 miles on a motorway at 70mph.

If the cost of petrol is 80p/l, how much do I spend on petrol on a given working day?

A £8.65

B £10.45

C £5.92

D £11.84

E £14.80

36. The problem is not that house prices are rising: a house is an asset, after all. The problem is the debt that sits behind it. To meet ever-rising prices, households are borrowing more. Average loan-to-income ratios are at an all-time high. This threatens to throttle the economy. Interest rate rises are likely: with more pay devoted to mortgage repayments, consumption is bound to slacken. That is bad news for firms, and, in turn, workers. A household debt hangover also reduces the funds that could be channelled towards productive investment. This slows GDP [Gross Domestic Product] now, and lowers potential too.

Which of the following best expresses the main conclusion of the argument above?

A The problem is not that house prices are rising, but that households are having to borrow more.

B Average loan-to-income ratios are at an all-time high.

C A high level of household indebtedness poses a risk to the economy.

D Interest rate rises are bad news for firms and workers.

E A high level of household indebtedness restrains productive investment.

37. To start a successful business, it is necessary to work hard. Therefore, if you start a business and work hard, your business will be successful.

Which of the following is the best statement of the flaw in the above argument?

A It ignores 'acts of God' such as floods and earthquakes.

B It assumes that people need to work hard to start a successful business.

C It overstates the importance of hard work in the success of a business.

D It ignores the fact that some people with a successful business never had to work hard.

E It assumes that hard work is a sufficient condition for the success of a business.

38. 'Mental disorder' is difficult to define. Generally speaking, mental disorders are conditions that involve either loss of contact with reality or distress and impairment. These experiences lie on a continuum of normal human experience, and so it is impossible to define the point at which they become pathological. _____ concepts such as schizophrenia, depression, and personality disorder listed in classifications of mental disorder may not in fact map onto any real or distinct disease entities; even if they do, the symptoms and clinical manifestations that define them are open to subjective interpretation.

Which of the following phrases, inserted in the blank space, most logically completes the above argument?

A   At the same time,

B   Furthermore,

C   That said,

D   Yet,

E   Similarly,

39. I have some 20p stamps and three times as many 50p stamps. The total value of the stamps is £10.20.

How many stamps do I have in total?

A   16

B   20

C   24

D   28

E   32

40. Mrs Jones has contracted a decorator to cover a wall in wallpaper.

To complete the job, the decorator is going to need 13 rolls of wallpaper at £25 per roll and 2 pots of glue at £6 per pot. He gets a 20% trade discount on the wallpaper and the glue.

He estimates that the job will take him 8 hours at £15 per hour plus VAT [Value-Added Tax] at 20%.

How much should he charge Mrs Jones in total?

A   £404.00

B   £413.60

C   £478.60

D   £416.00

E   £389.60

41. The hexagon below may be cut into six identical pieces.

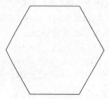

Which of the following pieces can be used six times (flips and rotations are allowed) to make up the hexagon?

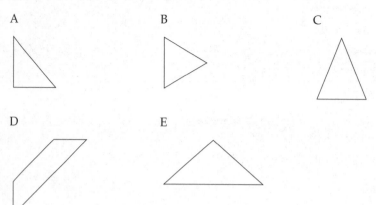

42. At peak times, standard class carriages on trains are so packed that most commuters cannot find a seat. This leaves even elderly or disabled people with little choice but to stand, not to mention the general discomfort of a closed and overcrowded space and the risk to public health that it poses. Meanwhile, First Class carriages are underutilised. Train operators could offer a better overall service if they converted First Class carriages to standard class, and did away with First Class altogether.

Which of the following, if true, would most weaken the above argument?

A   At off-peak times, First Class carriages are busier than standard class carriages.

B   Despite being underutilised at peak times, a First Class carriage raises considerably more revenue than a standard class carriage.

C   More people are travelling First Class than ever before.

D   Without First Class, some people would no longer travel by train.

E   Revenue raised by First Class helps to fund standard class carriages.

43. After five long years, the people of Europe must wish they could dispatch the entire political class to hellfire and torment. As it happens, the forthcoming ballot for elections to the European Parliament does not include that option, so a record number will probably abstain from voting. Many of those who do vote will back populists and extremists. Broadly anti-European parties may well take over a quarter of the seats. Anti-European parties in several member states are likely to win their highest vote ever. This will cause domestic political ructions, but it is above all an indictment of the European Union, a project that millions of voters have come to associate with hardship and failure.

Which of the following best expresses the main conclusion of the argument above?

A   Europeans are dissatisfied with their politicians.

B   A record number of people will abstain from voting in the forthcoming European elections.

C   Anti-European parties will do very well in the forthcoming European elections.

D   The success of anti-European parties in the forthcoming European elections will cause domestic political ructions.

E   The European Union is deeply unpopular.

44. The European Union should act only if and in so far as the objectives of a proposed action cannot be sufficiently achieved by the Member States, either at central level or at regional and local level, but can rather, by reason of the scale or effects of the proposed action, be better achieved at Union level.

Which one of the following best illustrates the principle underlying the above argument?

A   To boost competition and lower prices in the wireless services sector, the European Commission ought to establish a new European Telecom Markets Authority with the authority to over-rule national regulators and split up dominant market players.

B   The State should not confine itself to guaranteeing security and the rule of law; it should also guide individuals in all of their affairs and ensure, throughout their lives, that all of their needs are met.

C   Charity is best carried out at a local or individual level. By intervening directly, the State is depriving society of its responsibility, leading to a loss of human energies and an inordinate increase of costly public agencies.

D   Children should receive the same education regardless of where they live. That is why decisions about the education of our children should be left to the Ministry of Education, not to local school boards.

E   Capitalism should be maintained and encouraged because it provides the basis of calculation, in the shape of market prices, without which socialist enterprises would never be carried on, even within single branches of production or individual countries.

45. Every month, a telemarketing salesman makes £1,200 plus 2% on sales for that month.

Last month, he made £4,600.

What was the value of his sales?

A   £3,400

B   £17,000

C   £34,000

D   £170,000

E   £230,000

46. Some of the squares on a 4x4 board are marked with certain symbols, which may or may not be covered up by a circular counter. At one stage in the game, the board looks like this (all the circles represent counters which cover up the square that they occupy).

Which of the following represents a possible layout of the board (not necessarily viewed in the same direction as above)?

A

B

C

D

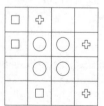

E

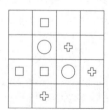

47. Greg and Priya are standing on either side of a block of buildings. The appearance of the buildings from above and the positions of Greg and Priya are shown below.

Priya

Greg

Greg sees this:

Which of the following **cannot** be the view that Priya sees?

A

B

C

D

E

48. My grandfather depends on my grandmother for his care. Unfortunately, she is now terminally ill. I fear that, when she dies, he will die too.

Which one of the following most closely parallels the kind of reasoning used in the passage above?

A   Grizzly bears depend on salmon for their diet. If the salmon die out, the bears will have to adapt their eating habits.'

B   You can only obtain a passport if you have an ID card. But you don't have an ID card, so you can't obtain a passport.

C   I can't ingest anything that contains nuts. The chocolate bar contains trace amounts of nuts, so I can't eat it.

D   If I accidentally ingest nuts, I have to give myself an adrenaline injection. If I don't receive the injection, I could die.

E   If I accidentally ingested nuts and did not receive an adrenaline injection, I could die. So I need to carry the injection with me at all times.

49. Economists agree that one reason for Britain's poor post-crisis productivity is that low wages encouraged firms to rely on human labour for low-skilled work, rather than investing in machines and software. Assuming that the economists are right, wage rises should start to reverse that trend, boosting investment and workers' productivity.

Which of the following is an underlying assumption of the argument above?

A   Firms want to control their costs as much as possible.

B   Low wages are good for employment.

C   Machines and software cannot replace high-skilled work.

D   Lack of investment increases workers' productivity.

E   Economists are always right.

50. Our intellect is like a sighted but lame man riding on the shoulders of a blind giant. Schopenhauer anticipates Freud by effectively equating the blind giant of will to our unconscious drives and fears, of which our conscious intellect may not be entirely or even mostly cognizant. For instance, the most powerful manifestation of will is the impulse for sex. Schopenhauer says that it is the will-to-life of the yet unconceived offspring that draws man and woman together in a delusion of lust and love. But with the task accomplished, their shared delusion fades away and they return to their 'original narrowness and neediness'.

Which of the following is a conclusion that can be drawn from the above argument?

A   The lame man represents our unconscious drives and fears.

B   The blind giant of will is mostly powerless.

C   Schopenhauer inspired the work of Freud.

D   We are mostly driven by our intellect.

E   We are mostly driven by unconscious forces.

Paper 1: (Answers)

1. **D** If all Freezians are Nachters, and all Nachters are Westerians, then all Freezians (which are a subset of Nachters) must also be Westerians. Some Nachters may not be Freezians, so A need not be true. By the same logic, some Westerians may not be Freezians, excluding B. All Nachters are Westerians, so C is patently false. Finally, while we know that no Esterian is a Nachter, and therefore not a Freezian either (since all Freezians are Nachters), we do not know whether Esterians are or can also be Westerians, eliminating E. If in doubt with a question like this, it can be helpful to sketch a Venn diagram to summarise the situation.

2. **C** Beware that, in this case, the conclusion actually appears before the premises; and one of the premises is hidden (i.e. it is an assumption).

    1. Each year for the past ten years, WH has received more votes than any other book... (Premise 1)

    2. Public opinion is a valid indicator of how good a book is. (Hidden Premise 2)

    3. Therefore, WH is the best book ever written in the English language. (Conclusion)

    A is merely a restatement of the conclusion. B is merely a restatement of the first premise. D and E, although true, do not connect the first premise to the conclusion.

3. **B** To summarise the argument, life expectancy is rising because more money is being spent on healthcare. However, it could be that life expectancy would have risen even if there had been no increase in health spending (B) owing to such factors as better nutrition, improved technology, and so on. The argument assumes that increased spending on healthcare is improving health outcomes, and that this in turn is increasing life expectancy. Instead, it could be that, despite the increased spending, the healthcare system is not delivering better health outcomes, or that better health outcomes are only one of several factors behind the increase in life expectancy. A, D, and E do not really encroach upon the argument. In particular, the fact that life expectancy at birth is rising (D) could also be linked to increased healthcare spending. That the healthcare system is sometimes criticised for delivering poor patient care (E) is perhaps inevitable, and need not mean that increased spending on healthcare is not improving overall health outcomes. Finally, the fact that healthier people can expect to live longer (C) serves, if anything, to strengthen the argument, which assumes this to be the case.

4. **A** You basically need to find the lowest common multiple (LCM) of 6, 9, and 24.

   One method is to list out multiples, starting with the highest number:

   24: 24, 48, **72**, 96

   6: 6, 12, 18, 24, 30, 36, 42, 48, 54, 60, 66, **72**, 78...

   9: 9, 18, 27, 36, 45, 54, 63, **72**, 81...

   The lowest common multiple is 72. So the next time that Eva, John, and Allan will all come in the same month is 72 months (6 years) from June 2014.

   Note that, if Allan comes every two years, the next time they all come will have to also be in June, so you can easily exclude D and E.

5. **A** The number of pupils reading both *Life of Pi* and *Siddharta* is 22. The total number of pupils reading *Life of Pi* is (10 + 22 + 8 + 26) 66. So the percentage of pupils reading *Life of Pi* who are also reading *Siddharta* is (22/66 x 100) 33.3%.

6. **D** The answer is not A as there is no change in TO between years 6 and 7.

   It is not B because TO falls between year 10 and 11.

   It is not C because TO does not go up quite that much between years 8 and 9.

   E is an inverse image of D.

7. **C** The argument is essentially that people cannot escape from making choices, because to escape from making choices is in itself to make a choice. From this, Sartre draws the momentous conclusion that man is condemned to be free. While A seems plausible, there is simply not enough evidence in the passage to conclude that *the vast majority* of people are living a lie. The passage merely states that 'people may pretend...' B can be rejected on similar grounds. There is nothing in the passage to suggest how common or uncommon self-deception actually is. D is merely a restatement of the assumption that 'people cannot pretend to themselves that they are not themselves'. Finally, E runs contrary to the passage. In particular, the passage states that 'a person may pretend to himself that he does not have the freedom to make choices, but to do so is in itself to make a choice'. In other words, people are condemned to make choices, 'man is condemned to be free'.

8. **D** The principle is that, even in matters of life and death, adults should be free to make their own choices, so long as their choices are truly their own, and so long as they fully understand the risks involved. A is about encouraging a choice, and B about imposing it. C argues that even young people (not necessarily adults) should be free to make their own choices, even if their choices are not truly their own and they do not fully understand the risks involved. E illustrates the converse principle that people should not be held accountable for their choices if their choices were not truly their own.

123

9. **E** Nagel argues: either death is an evil because it deprives us of life, or it is a mere blank because there is no subject left to experience the loss (C). So, if death is an evil, this is not in virtue of any positive attributes that it has (D), but because it deprives us of life (and life is intrinsically valuable). In order for Nagel to conclude that, if death is an evil, this is because it deprives us of life, he has to assume that life is intrinsically valuable (A). Don't confuse the conclusion with the assumption on the basis that the assumption comes after the conclusion. In the passage, B is used merely as another assumption or, perhaps more accurately, as a hypothesis.

10. **D** The long wall measures 5 x 2m. As each module measures 1.2 x 0.85m, you can fit a total of eight modules against the wall.

Trying to find the answer by working out the area of the wall and dividing by the area of the module (if you could do that in your head!) would be a mistake because the modules, being modules, cannot be broken down into smaller units.

Instead, you need to calculate how many modules fit lengthwise (5/1.2 = 4.17 = 4) and how many fit height-wise (2/0.85 = 2.35 = 2) and then multiply these two figures = 8.

Finally, given the answer options A to E, you should be able to see that 8 x 72 could only be D.

11. **C** In one month, Josefin will use (10 x 30) 300 peak and (30 x 30) 900 off-peak minutes.

The cost of doing so on £10 vouchers will be: (300 x 40p) + (900 x 10p) = 12,000p + 9,000p = 21,000p or £210

Answer B is using the £50 voucher.

Answer E is using the £5 voucher.

Answer D is adding the cost of the phone.

Answer A is forgetting to multiply by 30 days.

12. **E** Whereas you could create a quadrilateral (e.g. A), you could not possibly create a square. In answering this question, it could be useful to draw out the two triangles several times, each time overlapping them in a different way, for example, with one triangle upright and the other upside down, or one upright and the other on its side.

13. **A** The thrust of the argument is that, because Chardonnay has a very malleable profile, and because it is more widespread than any other grape variety (C), two Chardonnay wines can have strikingly little in common (B). Therefore, it is difficult to generalise about Chardonnay wines (A). Don't be thrown by the fact that the example comes after the conclusion, and, for this reason, mistake the example (E) for the conclusion. Given how widespread it is, one may be tempted to conclude that Chardonnay is a very successful grape variety (D), but this is not the particular conclusion of the passage.

14. **C** The essence of the passage is that the calculations imply that life is unlikely to have evolved on Mars. For example, it states that, 'Calculations suggest that the waters they formed would have been highly acidic. *That is bad enough for those who imagine them brim-full of bacteria. But they would also have been highly osmotic.'* A and B are no doubt true, but are not what the passage is driving at. D is simply a statement of fact contained in the passage. One can infer E from the passage, but, again, that is not what the passage is driving at.

15. **C** The passage is an example of arguing (fallaciously) for something by denigrating its alternatives. In this case, one issue is that there may be more than just two extreme alternatives. But even when there are just two alternatives, you cannot prove that one is good simply by arguing that the other is not; after all, they may both be equally bad. A recognises that Manchester United is merely one among several teams doing quite well. B is not merely damning the alternatives, but also offering evidence for the primacy of Manchester United. D is simply stating a fact: that Manchester United has scored more goals than the other three teams put together. E does not argue for the primacy of a particular team.

16. **B** Call the total distance that Jack travels x, and the total distance that Jill travels y. Call the amount of time that they travel before they meet t.

Since speed = distance/time, distance = speed x time

Therefore,

$x = 20t$

$y = 4t$

We know that $x + y = 6$, and so we solve.

$x + y = 6$

$20t + 4t = 6$

$24t = 6$

$t = 6/24 = 0.25$ hours = 15 minutes

17. C From the chart, the aircraft must fly a distance of 2,400km. It is flying at an average speed of 500 miles per hour, which is (500 x 1.6) 800 kilometres per hour. The time it takes to reach Moscow is (2,400km/800kmh) 3 hours, which is (3 x 60) 180 minutes. If you omitted to convert the speed from miles per hour to kilometres per hour, you would have answered (2,400/500) 4.8 hours or 288 minutes. If you had picked the wrong figure from the table, most likely 7,000, you would have answered (7,000/800) 8.75 hours or 525 minutes.

18. C Oxford is west of Thame, which is west of Aylesbury. High Wycombe is east of Thame, and west of Beaconsfield. Therefore Beaconsfield must be east of Oxford and Thame, but not necessarily Aylesbury. It can be helpful to draw a sketch.

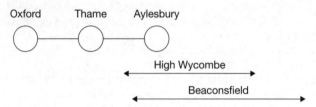

19. B The argument effectively assumes that specialisation improves quality (rather than productivity, C). However, in the case of research and teaching, this is not necessarily the case, with many academics gaining a teaching edge from their research and a research edge from their teaching. The passage is silent on which of research or teaching it considers more important (A). Finally, while D and E may complicate the implementation of the argument, they do not really touch upon its fundamental flaw.

20. A In sum: personhood depends on something more than just the brain. We are unable to grasp what this is because we tend to think of personhood as something concrete and tangible. *However* (but) this is not the kind of thing that personhood is.

21. C   The views are those of the ancient philosopher Epicurus. In essence, the argument is that, since anything that is good is so by virtue of the pleasure that it can procure, people ought to pursue those things that result in the greatest pleasure over time. The argument assumes that pleasure is the highest good (C). Another assumption of the argument is that people ought to pursue good things (which are good by virtue of the pleasure that they can procure), but that is not among the answer options. The passage does not assume that people are selfish (D); for example, it may be that helping others is very pleasurable (both to oneself and to others) and therefore that it ought to be pursued. In saying that people are unable to handle the hedonistic calculus, the passage may or may not be implying that people are stupid (E), but this would be more of an inference than an assumption. That the pursuit of pleasure is instinctive (B) is not an underlying assumption, not least because it is openly stated in the passage. Rather, this fact is used to buttress the argument—as is the fact that human beings can immediately feel that something is pleasurable (A).

22. D   Identify all those groups who moved into a larger house.

		Current house			
		≤ 2 bed	3 bed	≥ 4 bed	**Total**
Previous house	≤ 2 Bed	200	160	40	**400**
	3 Bed	80	200	80	**360**
	≥ 4 Bed	20	120	100	**240**
	Total	**300**	**480**	**220**	

(160 + 40 + 80) 280 people moved into a larger house. Therefore, the percentage trading up is 280/1000 or 28%.

23. D   Each team has to play every other team in its group twice.

–   Team A must play teams B, C, D, E, and F twice, i.e. 10 matches

–   Team B must then play teams C, D, E, and F twice, i.e. 8 matches

–   Team C must then play teams D, E, and F twice, i.e. 6 matches…

Thus, the total number of matches within each group = (10 + 8 + 6 + 4 + 2) 30

The total number of matches for both groups = (30 x 2) 60

Each team also plays each team in the other group once = (6 x 6) 36

Not forgetting that there is also one final.

So total number of matches = 60 + 36 + 1 = 97

24. C Call the number of 5p coins 'a' and the number of 10p coins 'b'.

a + b = 20

5a + 10b = 135

If a + b = 20, then a = 20 – b

So, substituting, 5(20 – b) + 10b = 135

100 – 5b + 10b = 135

100 + 5b =135

5b = 135 – 100

5b = 35

b = 35/5

b = 7

Since a + b = 20 and b = 7, a must equal (20 – 7) 13.

Alternatively, you can just work backwards from the answer options.

25. D The argument is that, rather than spending your resources on going to law school, you should spend them on starting a business, because starting a business will ultimately enable you to earn even more money. The argument assumes that you are only considering law school because studying law will enable you to make good money. But if most people who go to law school do so because they are genuinely interested in the law (D), then that assumption is false. Even if A and B were true, the argument would not be undermined. In particular, what you can do (or are ready to do) and what you should do are not one and the same thing. The passage already takes into account that many new businesses fail (C). The fact that a large minority of people who go to law school end up starting their own business (E) arguably strengthens rather than detracts from the argument.

26. C According to the passage, death not only deprives us of life, but also casts its shadow upon us while we are still living (C). A is only a partial statement of the conclusion of the passage. B effectively says the same thing as A. It is true that the passage states that our fear of death is mostly unconscious (D), but this is hardly its conclusion. E goes one step further in stating that it is our unconscious fear of death that holds us back from exercising choice and freedom; but this merely explains or elaborates upon the conclusion of the passage by telling us *how* death mars our life.

27. **A** As only 32% of lawyers work as barristers, more lawyers must work as solicitors than as barristers, making 1 true. We are told that 32% of lawyers work as barristers *at least some of the time*; however unlikely, it is just possible that none of them work as barristers *all of the time*, making 2 false. The same reasoning also applies to 3: although 32% of lawyers work as barristers at least some of the time, we cannot be 100% sure, on the basis of the limited information provided in the passage, that any of them spend more time working as barristers than as solicitors.

28. **D** Depth rises slowly at first, then rapidly, then slowly again. So the cross-section must be wider at the top and bottom compared to the middle. Admittedly, D is a very unusual shape for any cistern—but there you are.

29. **A** Linda sold the shares for $(5{,}000 + (20/100 \times 5{,}000))$ £6,000 the first time.

    She then re-invested this sum into the shares, which rose by a further 45% $(45/100 \times 6{,}000 = £2{,}700)$ before she sold them again for a total of $(6{,}000 + 2{,}700)$ £8,700.

    So she made an overall profit of $(8{,}700 - 5{,}000)$ £3,700 or $(3{,}700/5{,}000 \times 100)$ 74%.

30. **D** The remaining people in the sample (those who went on holiday outside Europe) equate to $(100 - 30 - 25 - 20)$ 25% of the sample. This amounts to $(8 + 6 + 5)$ 19 people. Therefore, the number of people who participated in the survey is $100/25 \times 19 = 76$

31. **E** The condensed form of the argument is as follows. Many novels that are tightly plotted have been unsuccessful. At the same time, some novels that are loosely plotted have been very successful. Therefore, to be successful, all novels should be loosely plotted. Of course, loosely plotted novels can be successful for reasons other than being loosely plotted: for example, they may feature an inspiring protagonist or be rich in imagination. A, B, C, and D are all more or less true, but, out of that list, are not the *best expression* of the flaw in the argument. Perhaps a more fundamental flaw is that the fact that many novels that are tightly plotted have been unsuccessful need not necessarily mean that tightly plotted novels are not more successful overall.

32. **C** The form of the argument is: if all A's are B, and all C's are A's, then all C's are B. The five options are all valid arguments. D and E are the same form of argument: if all A's are B's, and all B's are C's, then all A's are C's. A takes the form of: if X is a Y, and all Y's are A, then X is A. B takes the form of: if the X's are Y's, and all Y's are A, then the X's are A.

33. E This is the apocryphal Paradox of the Court. Having learnt the wily ways of his master, Euathlus retorted that if he won the case he would not have to pay, and if Protagoras won the case, he still would not have to pay, because he still would not have won a case! The solution to the paradox is still debated to this day. One could argue that Protagoras could not possibly win the case (D), but, even if that were true, his argument would be untouched. The same reasoning also applies to A, B, and C. For example, Protagoras' argument turns on Euathlus either losing or winning the case, so the argument (if not the case) would still stand if Euathlus engaged a lawyer to represent him (B).

34. D The crew takes the 07:15 flight to Madrid, arriving at 09:15, and flies back to Zürich on the 10:15 flight, arriving at 12:15.

It then flies back out to Madrid on the 14:30 flight, arriving at 16:30, and back to Zürich on the 17:20 flight, arriving at 19:20.

So the total time from take-off on the first flight to landing on the last flight of the day is 12 hours 5 minutes.

35. D It's important to be constantly aware that John must throw the die four times. A score of 10 points could be made up by any combination of (5, 3, 1, 1) and any combination of (3, 3, 3, 1). There are no other possibilities. A score of 12 points could be made up of any combination of (5, 5, 1, 1), (3, 3, 3, 3), or (5, 3, 3, 1). A score of 14 points could be made up by any combination of (5, 5, 3, 1) and any combination of (5, 3, 3, 3). A score of 18 points could be made up by any combination of (5, 5, 5, 3). On the other hand, a score of 15 cannot be arrived at with four throws. It could be arrived at with three throws of 5, but then there would need to be another throw which would add on either 1, 3, or 5. Two throws of 5 and one throw of 3 would bring us to 13, but the fourth throw cannot be 2. One throw of 5 and three throws of 3 would be one short.

36. A The key is to find the limiting element.

There are only 200 guidance leaflets in the warehouse, meaning that at most 200 kits can be assembled.

200 kits would require (200 x 20) 4,000 washproof plasters. But there are only 2,000 washproof plasters, so the highest number of kits that can be assembled is (2,000/20) 100.

100 kits would require 400 triangular bandages, 600 safety pins, 800 sterile dressings, and 1,000 moist wipes—happily, these are all in stock.

As there are 12 kits per carton, the maximum number of cartons that can be dispatched from the warehouse is (100/12) 8.33 i.e. 8.

37. **C** The form of the argument is as follows. X is happening. To stop X, Y must happen. Unless X is stopped, Z will happen. *Therefore, to stop Z, Y must happen.* X is population growth, Y is expanding family planning options in developing countries, and Z is environmental disaster. The passage clearly states that population growth can be curbed, so A is false. B is most likely true, but cannot be concluded on the basis of the information provided in the passage. D and E are merely restatements of a premise in the argument, not the conclusion to which the argument is building.

38. **B** The assumption that courage is always a fine and noble thing is used to demonstrate that the second man, whose behaviour is more foolish and therefore the opposite of fine and noble, is not in fact the more courageous. Although the author clearly thinks that most people have a mistaken notion of courage, he does not assume that whatever people think must be wrong (A). The author does assume that children and animals have no sense, but this is explicitly stated and is not central to his argument (C). The example from Homer merely 'suggests' (rather than 'proves' or 'demonstrates') that courage amounts not to blind recklessness (D). Finally, E is merely a succinct restatement of the conclusion of the passage. The passage is adapted from Plato's *Laches*.

39. **C** Correlation does not imply causation. While there is indeed an association between bipolar disorder and creativity (C), this need not mean that one leads to the other (A, B). For example, it may be that people with bipolar disorder are more attracted to careers in the arts that value and exercise creativity. The passage merely says that people with bipolar disorder and creative people share certain temperamental tendencies, not that they all have similar temperaments (D). Finally, while it is true that not all people with bipolar disorder are creative (E), there is nothing in the passage to support this claim.

40. **D** The top left box represents the number of candidates (110) who passed both the mock exam and the actual exam. The top right box represents the number of candidates (10) who passed the mock exam but failed the actual exam. The bottom left box represents the number of candidates (50) who failed the mock exam but passed the actual exam. Finally, the bottom right box represents the number of candidates (70) who failed both the mock exam and the actual exam. The candidates who had their results correctly predicted by their mock exam results are those who passed both the mock exam and the actual exam (110) and those who failed both the mock exam and the actual exam (70) = 180. $180/(110 + 70 + 50 + 10 = 240) = 75\%$

41. **E** When it is a quarter past three, the minute hand is exactly on 3, while the hour hand is one-quarter of the way from 3 to 4. The distance between 3 to 4 represents 1/12 of the circumference of the clock face. The clock face comprises $360°$, so the angle between 3 and 4 o'clock is $(360/12) = 30°$. One quarter of this is $(30/4)$ $7.5°$.

42. **E**   If people who are predisposed to developing schizophrenia are also predisposed to smoking cannabis, then the link between smoking cannabis and developing schizophrenia is probably not causal. The other answer options do not undermine the potential for a causal link between smoking cannabis and developing schizophrenia. In other words, even if these options were true, it could still be the case that smoking cannabis increases the risk of developing schizophrenia.

43. **E**   In a nutshell, the argument is that people who have suffered traumatic early life experiences may in later life compensate for negative feelings by seeking out achievement and success. Of the five options, evidence of an association between above average achievement and success and traumatic early life experiences (E) most strengthens the argument. D also strengthens the argument but not as much as E, because low self-esteem has many causes including but not limited to traumatic early life experiences. A, B, and C tend to weaken the argument. A arguably does not even touch the argument, as one does not need to have the memory of the trauma to suffer from its effects.

44. **D**   Quick solution: as Mary started out heavier than John, and John lost more weight than Mary, Mary cannot possibly be lighter than John.

45. **E**

   - 16 squares making up the large square (1) = 17

   - 4 small squares making up the two central squares (2) = 10

   - 9 2x2 squares = 9

   - 4 3x3 squares = 4

   Total = (17 + 10 + 9 + 4) 40

46. **A**   According to the passage, we impose structures such as space and time onto the world of appearances, and it is through these structures that we apprehend the individual things that make up the world as we know it. It follows that the world as it appears to us is a product of the structures that we impose upon it, and therefore a product of the kind of organism that we are (A). To go on and conclude that individual material things do not exist (B) is a step too far. Similarly, the passage is silent on whether or not our experiencing self is itself an object in the world of appearances (C). The passage states that 'the world of appearances is the world that we perceive through our senses', suggesting that the world as it is cannot be perceived through our senses. Nonetheless, we cannot know this for sure, and, in any case, there may well be other, extra-sensorial, ways of apprehending the world as it actually is (D). Finally, we all know for a fact that our senses can be mistaken (E), but this cannot be concluded solely on the basis of the information provided in the passage.

47. **A**   The best statement of the flaw in the argument is that it employs an exceptional case to reject a general rule. True, there may be some rare circumstances in which it is best not to (immediately) repay a debt, but this does not mean that repaying a debt is wrong in principle. While the material introduced is exceptional, it is not strictly speaking irrelevant (B). Neither is the argument circular (supported by its own conclusion, C), as in, for example, 'We should reject the idea that is just to repay what is owed because to repay what is owed is wrong in principle.' D and E merely qualify or mitigate the example, without however pointing to the actual flaw in the argument.

48. **E**   Since the cost of a house burglary, car burglary, and theft are in a ratio of 100:10:1, divide every number in the theft column by 100 by moving the decimal point two places to the left, and divide every number in the car burglary column by 10 by moving the decimal point one place to the left. This weights the events according to their cost to the insurance company. Lastly, tally up the three numbers to obtain a figure that is proportional to the overall cost in that month.

	Theft	Car burglary	House burglary	**Total**
January	2.30	6.0	30	38.3
February	2.40	6.2	28	36.6
March	2.55	7.0	28	37.55
April	3.10	7.5	24	34.6
May	3.65	8.0	20	31.65
June	4.50	6.0	16	26.5
July	5.00	5.0	10	20
August	5.22	5.0	22	32.22
September	3.50	6.5	14	24
October	3.20	7.0	22	32.2
November	2.36	7.0	24	33.36
December	2.50	6.0	30	38.5

Quick solution: you can see just by eyeballing the numbers that the most expensive month is going to be either December or January, so you only have to apply the above method to these two months.

49. E We know that:

A + 2T = £100 &

2A + 7T = £275

If A + 2T = £100, then A = £100 - 2T

Substituting into the second equation,

2 (100 - 2T) + 7T = 275

200 - 4T + 7T = 275

200 + 3T = 275

3T = 275 - 200 = 75

T = 75/3 = £25

Therefore A = £50

There is also a much quicker method: if you assume that D is true, you can quickly work out that an atlas is £50 and a textbook is £25.

Remember that you can often work backwards from the answer options.

50. A This is a distance time graph, not a speed time graph. So when the driver starts going back home, the gradient will turn negative i.e. the answer cannot be B. E may be the most elegant of the lines, but it fails to account for the driver's various changes in speed on his way out and, presumably, also on his way back home (as he hits town again and has to slow down). C fails to account for the slowing down at the road works. D fails to account for the stopping at the road works.

Paper 2: (Answers)

1. **E** As things stand, America has better military equipment and more experienced military personnel than China. This need not necessarily mean that American forces are very well equipped (A). Even Chinese commanders acknowledge that China will not be able to match American hard power until 2050 at the earliest. Moreover, America has many more close allies than China and Russia, which, overall, increases its military might. Thus, one can safely conclude that America will remain the dominant power for the foreseeable future (E). One cannot conclude that, after 2050, China will become the dominant power (B), because being able to do something and actually doing it are two very different things (and, of course, the Chinese commanders could be wrong in their assessment). Although one can infer that America and China are rivals for military supremacy, and might one day be enemies, this need not imply that they are currently enemies (D). Similarly, although the passage does speak of China and Russia in the same breath, it remains silent about whether or not they are allies (C).

2. **D** The principal problem with the study is that it could well be the daily exercise that explained the weight loss. If, however, the women in the study exercised regularly before entering the study, it becomes much more likely that it was indeed the dietary change (rather than the exercise) that led to the weight loss.

3. **A** We are looking for the smallest number of male students who are going straight into house jobs. So we have to assume that all those students who are going into research posts (20) and other jobs are male (10), leaving just 20 male students going straight into house jobs. Next, we have to assume that all the 15 international students are males going straight into house jobs, leaving only 5 positions for home students.

4.   **E**   If a month contains 31 days, it contains at least four of each day of the week (4 x 7 = 28), with three consecutive days left over.

   If the month contains five Mondays, one of those three leftover days must be a Monday.

   - If it is the first leftover day, the other two leftover days are Tuesday and Wednesday (and the month started on a Monday).

   - If it is the second, the other two days are Sunday and Tuesday (and the month started on a Sunday).

   - If it is the third, the other two days are Saturday and Sunday (and the month started on a Saturday).

July						
Su	Mo	Tu	We	Th	Fr	Sa
	1	2	3	4	5	6
7	8	9	10	11	12	13
14	15	16	17	18	19	20
21	22	23	24	25	26	27
28	29	30	31			

5.   **C**   It is helpful, for each treasure hunter, to sketch out (or visualise) the perimeter in which the treasure could be located. The treasure will be at the intersection of the three areas. Remember that the perimeters are circular rather than square.

6.   **A**   The passage states that, *most of the time*, a person's actions are determined, and that a 'window of freedom' is *more or less uncommon*. On reading the passage, it seems plausible that most people never exercise free will, but this cannot be formally concluded solely on the basis of the information provided (B). C, D, and E can all be inferred from the information provided, but neither option is the main conclusion of the passage, which is, ultimately, about how free actions can occur given that most actions are determined. The passage is an expression of the 'effort of thought' theory of free will.

7.   **C**   Evidence of association is not evidence of causation. People who drink red wine in moderate amounts tend to be better off than average. They are more likely to sit down for their meals, and so to enjoy better nutrition and lower levels of stress. Perhaps they are also more sociable and happier. Thus, it is not the wine that is making them healthier, but other factors in their diets or lifestyles (C). A, B, and E are all true, but do not directly impact on the argument. D may or may not be true, but, even if it is, that need not mean that the research is bogus. In any case, the truth or falsity of D does not impact on the actual dynamics of the argument.

8. **C** This is a very difficult question. The argument is essentially that people employ the manic defence in a whole range of forms or situations so as to fill their time and thoughts with pseudo-purposeful activities and thereby block out feelings of helplessness and despair, which is their real if subconscious purpose. The argument rests on the assumption that the process is subconscious; by bolstering that assumption, C most strengthens the argument.

9. **C**

    – Solid lines: 2,000m x 2 = 4,000m, 4,000m/(5m/L) = 800L

    – Dashed lines: 2,000m/(20m/L) = 100L

    – Curved arrows: 8 x 3L = 24L

    – Total = 924L

    – Number of drums of paint required = 924/5 = 184.5

10. **D** There are 37 companies with a TO of £1M or less.

    There are 50 companies included in the survey.

    37/50 x 100 = 74%

11. **D** The size of the office is 5.2 x 6.7m, and the size of the lobby is 3.6 x 4.4m. So that both pieces can be cut out, the offcut piece will have to be at least 5.2 x (6.7 + 3.6)m, i.e. 5.2 x 10.3m. Of course, it could be larger, but that would leave more spare carpet behind and be more expensive. For comparison, the five areas (from A to E) are 47.3 (too small), 58.96, 64.32, 53.56, and 57.72.

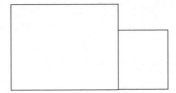

12. **B** The argument is as follows. The legalisation of prostitution leads to an overall increase in the demand for prostitution; but, because customers favour legal over trafficked prostitutes, the net effect is to reduce human trafficking. The [incorrect] assumption here is that, in terms of human trafficking, the effect of the increase in demand for prostitution does not outweigh the effect of customers favouring legal over trafficked prostitutes. A is merely a restatement of the conclusion of the argument. C, D, and E are assumptions of sorts, but overlie rather than *underlie* the argument.

13. **D** This is a very hard question, so, if you got it right, you will probably do very well on the critical thinking component of the TSA! The argument is essentially that, as people do not regard non-existence as an evil, if death is an evil, this is not because it involves non-existence, but because it deprives us of life. A, B, and C all undermine this argument and therefore weaken rather than strengthen it. A and B undermine the idea that death can be 'suffered', and thereby that it is an evil. Given that people 'do not regard the long period of time before they were born as an evil', the proposition that people regard the time after they are dead no differently to the time before they are born (C) similarly undermines the idea that death is an evil. This leaves only D and E. D effectively states that a person can suffer an evil even though he is dead, and can therefore 'suffer' death by being deprived of life. E is more an assumption of the argument than an additional piece of information.

14. **A** Sum all rows and columns and identify which two are incorrect. The incorrect entry is at their intersection. Alternatively, just sum the units place for each column and take it from there.

15. **C** Each team has to play each other team once.

    – Team A must play teams B, C, D, E, F, G, H

    – Team B must then play teams C, D, E, F, G, H

    – Team C must then play teams D, E, F, G, H…

    Thus, the total number of matches within each group = (7 + 6 + 5 + 4 + 3 + 2 + 1) 28

    Total number of matches for all groups = (28 x 4) 112

    Number of quarter-finals = 4

    Number of semi-finals = 2

    Number of finals = 1

    Total number of all matches = (112 + 4 + 2 + 1) 119

16. **A**

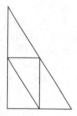

17. D Let's look at this argument again:

1. Each year for the past ten years, WH has received more votes than any other book... (Premise 1)

2. Public opinion is a valid indicator of how good a book is. (Hidden Premise 2)

3. Therefore, WH is the best book ever written in the English language. (Conclusion)

All the answer options present potential problems with the argument, but D attacks the second (hidden) premise most directly and is therefore the best statement of the flaw in the argument.

18. E The argument is that the effectiveness of antidepressants has been greatly exaggerated. The bulk of the passage presents evidence to shore up this argument. The effect size of the antidepressants was very small for all but very severe cases of depression. Moreover (in addition), this increased effect size was attributed not to an increase in the effect of the antidepressants, but to a decrease in their placebo effect—supporting the argument that the effectiveness of antidepressants has been greatly exaggerated. This second proposition adds to the first; it does not derive from it (A, C), compare to it (D), or qualify it (B).

19. B The hidden assumption is that people who are gifted in the arts (necessarily) have very good taste.

20. D The minute hand must take an hour to go round the clock face, even though it travels four times as fast down to 6 as it does back to 12. So the ratio of the time it takes to get from 12 to 6 to the time it takes to get from 6 to 12 is 1:4.

It will take $1/(1 + 4)$ of an hour for it to get down to 6, which is $(1/5 \times 60)$ 12 minutes. So the correct time when the clock shows half past one is 12 minutes past one.

21. D After one year, the house would have been worth (400,000 + £40,000) £440,000.

After two years, it would have been worth (440,000 + 44,000) £484,000.

After three years, it would have been worth (484,000 + 48,400) £532,400.

If you had had a calculator, you could have inputted $400,000 \times 1.10^3$.

139

22. E The shape consists of a different kind of L-shape table (right). It could not be made with the shape in the question.

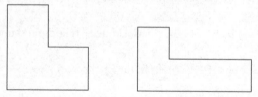

23. E Amanda and Adam are effectively using the shopping list/notebook as a security to make sure that any unusual or exceptional items have not been forgotten.

24. C The argument is essentially that, because the underlying nature of reality cannot be observed through sense experience, the underlying nature of reality is unknowable. This relies on two underlying assumptions: first, that nature is not as it appears (but this is not one of the five options), and, second, that knowledge of the underlying nature of reality can only be gained through sense experience (C). The argument does assume that sense experience is not objective (A), that the underlying nature of reality cannot be observed through sense experience (B), and that knowledge of the underlying nature of reality cannot be gained through sense experience (D), but these are explicit rather than underlying assumptions. Also, A does not underlie the argument—in other words, the argument would still have stood even if A had not been assumed. Finally, the passage does not seem or need to assume that true belief is equivalent to knowledge—all the opposite, in fact, as it states that 'the *best that can be hoped for* is true belief', implying that true belief is in some way inferior to knowledge.

25. B The government aims to improve access to university education for young people from disadvantaged backgrounds. Yet it has implemented a system of loans that is thought to deter poorer students from going to university. Therefore, the government's action goes against its aim. C states the opposite, so is clearly false. However likely A and D may seem, they cannot be concluded from the limited information in the passage. The passage merely states that students from poorer families are more likely to be deterred from going to university by the prospect of debt. This certainly need not imply that they are less ambitious (E).

26. **B**

   - 2012: 100%

   - 2013: 60% (-40%)

   - 2014: 15% (-75%)

   - 2015: 100/15 = 6.67

   - 667%

27. **B**   Before you panic at the sight of so many large numbers, notice the handy percent column at the far right. Identify the country with the largest population as a percentage of the total Eurozone population. Unsurprisingly, this is Germany, with 24.6% of the total Eurozone population. The next most populous country is France, with 19.6% of the total Eurozone population. 24.6 + 19.6 = 44.2, which is still short of 50%. So find the next most populous country, which is Italy, with 18.3% of the total Eurozone population. That extra 18.3% easily carries us over the 50% line. To be precise, Germany, France, and Italy together account (or accounted in 2012) for a whopping 62.5% of the Eurozone population.

28. **A**

   The closing price on 13th May is 36p per share.

   There are 250m shares in issue.

   Therefore, the value of the company is (250m x £0.36) = £90m

29. **D**   The argument is that 'altruistic' acts are in fact selfish, at the very least because they relieve unpleasant feelings and lead to pleasant ones. However, the fact that such acts relieve unpleasant feelings and lead to pleasant ones need not necessarily mean that they are selfish. An act should not be written off as selfish simply because it includes an often inevitable element of self-interest. In particular, it may be that the 'selfish' element is accidental, or, if not accidental, secondary, or, if neither accidental nor secondary, undetermining. A is simply a restatement of the conclusion. B, while more nuanced, does not state the flaw in the argument. C and E approach D, but, unlike D, do not explicitly state the flaw in the argument.

30. **D**   In short: distinguishing between social phobia and shyness is difficult and controversial. Some say that social phobia does not exist. But (however) social phobia differs from shyness in that it starts at a later age and is more severe and debilitating. The second sentence qualifies the first. 'In contrast' (E) tends to be used for a diametric opposition.

31. **A** The basic structure of the argument appears to be: A implies B. A. Therefore B. But in fact the two A's are not equivalent. The first A refers to human laws, whereas the second A refers to natural laws. So the underlying structure of the argument is: A implies B. C. Therefore B. This is the fallacy of equivocation, in which a key term or phrase is used in an ambiguous way, with one meaning in one part of the argument and another meaning in another part of the argument. A clearer example is: A feather is light. What is light cannot be dark. Therefore, a feather cannot be dark (A). Light is used to mean both 'light in weight' and 'bright'. B is a simple, valid argument. C is an example of a false dilemma (or fallacy of the excluded middle) in which limited options are considered when there are in fact more options. D is an example of exclusive premises, invalid because both premises are negative. As you may recall, no valid conclusion can ever be derived from two negative premises. Finally, E is an example of affirming the consequent (or converse error). The argument essentially fails to recognise that there can be more than one way of skinning a cat.

32. **E** If Dr Pideritt bought 36 copies, he would receive a 25% discount.

    So he would pay (36 x 25) £900 x 3/4 = £675

    If he bought 40 copies, he would receive a 40% discount.

    So he would pay (40 x 25) £1000 x 3/5 = £600

    He would therefore save (675-600) £75.

33. **B** We know that the number of pupils on the playground cannot be a multiple of 2—in other words, that it has to be an odd number. We also know that it is not a multiple of 3, 4, 5, or 6. 57, 69, 87, and 93 are all multiples of 3. Don't be intimidated by the look of the question; you can quickly arrive to the answer by simple elimination.

34. **A** A and B are very similar, but B fails to represent the fall in rainfall from December to January. C is the inverse of A.

35. **C** The argument is, essentially, that people should mow their lawn in winter because it is beneficial to do so. If, in addition to the benefits in the passage, mowing in winter also helps in the removal of leaf litter and debris, then this strengthens the case for mowing in winter. The fact that people need more exercise (B) also strengthens the argument, but mowing the lawn is not the best way of getting exercise. That grass stops growing when the air temperature falls below about 5°C (A), if anything, weakens the argument, and the same is also true of D and E.

36. A The passage basically consists in a series of 'examples of values that are far from timeless and universal'. From this, it is legitimate to conclude that [some values] are not timeless and universal (A). To conclude D or E on the basis of the passage alone would be a step too far. We may well agree that morals have progressed since the decline of the British Empire (C), but there is nothing in the passage to warrant this conclusion. Finally, while it can be inferred that the values held by a society can change very fast (B), this is not the best expression of the conclusion of the passage, which serves to illustrate the point that 'values are far from timeless and universal'.

37. E The fallacy of accident is committed when a general rule (the speed limit) is applied to a situation in which it was not intended to apply (a medical emergency). The fallacy suggests that there can be no exceptions to a general rule or principle. If applied to the letter, the principle that it is wrong to hurt animals would prevent us from controlling pests such as termites or rats (E). This is different from merely upholding the principle (C, D) but presumably allowing some exceptions for e.g. pests. A is not equivalent to E because watching live football is not an extraordinary circumstance. Severe diarrhoea (B) is more of an extraordinary circumstance, but in this case the driver did agree to bend the rule.

38. E John is older than Sarah and Sarah is younger than Freddy

- J/F > S

Freddy is older than John, but younger than Mary

- F > J > S
- M > F > J > S

39. C For a 200-page book, the cost of typesetting is (40/100 x 4,000) £1,600. For a 300-page book this goes up by (25/100 x 1600) £400 to £2,000.

For a 200-page book, the cost of printing is (50/100 x 4,000) £2,000. For a 300-page book, this goes up by (15/100 x 2,000) £300 to £2,300.

The cost of cover design remains (10/100 x 4,000) £400.

So the total cost of publishing a 300-page book is (2,000 + 2,300 + 400) £4,700.

40. C

- 16 unitary triangles in the large triangle (1) = 17
- 6 upright triangles consisting of four unitary triangles = 6
- 1 inverted triangle consisting of four unitary triangles = 1
- 3 triangles consisting of nine unitary triangles = 3

Total = (17 + 6 + 1 + 3) 27

41. C In short, the argument is that the distress caused to some people by living in a modern society is often expediently labeled as a mental disorder. This can be counterproductive as it can prevent the source of their distress from being identified and addressed. If depression is very rarely witnessed in traditional or historical societies (C), this bolsters the contention that the condition is in fact a manifestation of the distress of living in a modern society. A and B undermine this claim by suggesting that depression is instead a biological disorder of the brain. D and E do strengthen the argument, but not nearly so much as C, which does most to bolster the assumption that the condition is not in fact a mental disorder.

42. A The passage is an extract from *I Drink Therefore I Am*, by the British philosopher Roger Scruton. The argument is essentially that the drink problem in British cities stems from cultural impoverishment. This assumes that there was once a time when people were more cultured, and, as a result, did not have a drink problem—or, at least, not so much of a drink problem. Scruton does assume D and E, but, strictly speaking, these assumptions do not underlie his argument. He does not necessarily assume B and C. Note that it is not clear whether Scruton assumes that young people who drink primarily drink wine, or would drink wine if they knew better.

43. D The major and minor premises are universal affirmatives, as is the conclusion.

44. B Mr Sanders' fee for 14 hours of tuition would be (50 x 14) £700.

As Mrs Patel offers an extra 40 minutes per 4 hours booked, John would only have to book 12 hours to receive 14 hours of tuition (since 12/4 = 3 and 3 x 40 mins = 2 hours). 12 hours with Mrs Patel would cost (60 x 12) £720.

So John would save (720-700) £20.

45. C Note that, in this particular case, the triangles are right-angled triangles. In answering the question, it could be useful to draw out the two triangles several times, each time overlapping them in a different way, for example, with one triangle upright and the other upside down, or one upright and the other on its side.

46. B The argument is that, because 'dyslexia' lacks meaning and educational value (C, D), it should be ditched (B). This would avoid undermining and distressing children and free up resources to help them read (A, D).

47. C The argument is utilitarian in that it holds that the proper or best course of action is the one that, on the balance of probabilities, maximises total benefit. C in contrast is deontological in that it holds that the proper or best course of action is the one that is morally required, regardless of its potential consequences. The other main ethical framework (not covered in this question) is virtue ethics.

48. A   The major premise is a universal negative, the minor premise is a particular affirmative, and the conclusion is a particular negative.

49. C   40 people are neither self-employed nor in online retailing, leaving 210 people who are in one or other or both.

We know that 180 of these are self-employed, leaving (210–180) 30 who are in online retailing *and* not self-employed.

As there are 50 people in online retailing, that leaves (50–30) 20 people who are both self-employed and in online retailing.

50. A   It can be very helpful to sketch the initial diagram on a piece of paper, which you can then rotate around and compare to the answer options. Focus on the spatial relationship between the three visible symbols and take it from there.

Paper 3: (Answers)

1. **D** The passage contains a lot of distracting material, making it more challenging to extract the bare bones of the argument. The essence of the argument is as follows. The distinctive function of human beings is their capacity to reason. Therefore, the Supreme Good for human beings is to lead a life that enables them to exercise and to develop their reason. The underlying assumption or hidden premise is: the Supreme Good for a thing is for that thing to exercise its distinctive function (D). A is a restatement of an example cited in the passage. The passage merely states that even animals can enjoy amusement and pleasure. This need not entail that human beings should not pursue amusement or pleasure (B); in any case, this is certainly not an underlying assumption of the argument. That the capacity to reason is unique to human beings (C) is explicitly stated, and, as with B, is peripheral to the argument. Finally, E is a restatement of the conclusion.

2. **E** The author of the passage effectively dismisses the fanciful theories on the grounds that a more simple and ordinary explanation is available. In other words, the author has applied Occam's Razor, the principle of parsimony (*lex parsimoniae*) which states that, among competing hypotheses, the one with the fewest assumptions ought to be upheld. A is merely a restatement of the author's conclusion. B is explicitly stated in the first sentence of the passage. C, however true, is not, in this case, an underlying assumption but an unwarranted conclusion. The author of the passage may or may not believe in the truth of D, but, in any case, it is not the basis on which he or she dismisses the fanciful theories.

3. **D** The argument is, essentially, that the scheme will not lead to an overall fall in the insurance premiums of young motorists because the penalty for bad driving (up to 15 per cent) is greater than the reward for good driving (up to 11 per cent). However, if the vast majority of young motorists under the scheme drive responsibly (D), then the penalty for bad driving will only apply to a few, while everyone else will enjoy a discount. A, B, and E also weaken the argument, but not nearly as much as D. C actually strengthens the argument.

4. **D** The surface area of the first vineyard is (100 x 40) 4,000m².

   The density of vines is (1,440/4,000) 0.36 vines/m².

   The surface area of the second vineyard is (300 x 80) 24,000m².

   So the number of vines in the second vineyard is (24,000 x 0.36) 8,640.

   A quicker way is to see that the second vineyard is three times as long and twice as wide as the first, and therefore six times the surface area.

5. **B** Relative speed is (720-500) 220km/h.

With relative speed, the situation is the same as if the missile were standing still.

Speed = distance/time

Time = distance/speed

Time = 110/220 = 0.5h = 30mins

6. **A** The ratio of Eloise's speed on the ski lift to her speed on the ski run is 5:20 or 1:4.

So, given that the ski lift and the ski run are the same length, the ratio of the time that she spends on the ski lift to the time that she spends on the ski run is 4:1.

30/(4 + 1) = 6 minutes per unit of ratio

So she spends (4 x 6) 24 minutes on the ski lift, and (1 x 6) 6 minutes on the ski run.

Skiing at 20km/h for 6 minutes (1/10 of an hour), she will cover (20 x 1/10) 2km.

You can check this answer by calculating the distance covered on the ski lift: 5 x 24/60 = 2

7. **E** One cannot conclude that all psychopaths have a lot in common (A) because the passage is not categorical and absolute but hypothetical and relative in this regard, stating merely that 'it may be that highly successful and disturbed psychopaths have more in common than first meets the eye'. Similarly, one cannot conclude that most highly successful people are psychopaths (B) on the basis that 'compared to mentally disordered criminal offenders…. high-level executives were more likely to have one of three personality disorders'. For example, it could be that only a minority of high-level executives had a personality disorder, or that high-level executives are not representative of successful people as a whole. Also, the passage says only that 'high-level executives were more likely to have *one of three* personality disorders', not that they are more likely to have a personality disorder overall (C). It is much more difficult to decide between D and E, but D seems more like an intermediary conclusion which then enables the author of the passage to conclude E. To make things even more difficult, E is not explicitly stated, but implied by the William James quotation.

8. **C**   In essence, the passage argues that, because people with debilitating disorders have fewer children, genes for debilitating disorders usually pass out of the population over time; as this has not happened for bipolar disorder, the genes for bipolar disorder must be conferring an important adaptive or evolutionary advantage that promotes their survival in the population. Both A and B weaken the argument by undermining its premises. D also weakens the argument, as it suggests that carriers of the genes for bipolar disorder do not benefit from any particular adaptive or evolutionary advantage. Both E and C strengthen the argument; whereas C is a trend, E could just be an outlier, and so C most strengthens the argument. As an aside, it seems that only three medical conditions are more common in higher than lower socioeconomic groups: bipolar disorder, obsessive-compulsive disorder, and gout.

9. **C**   The form of the argument in the passage is as follows: Either X or Y. Not X. Therefore Y.

10. **D**   As chair 15 and chair 92 cross each other, there are (92–15) 77 chairs ahead of (or above) them including one of either chair 15 or 92, let's say chair 92.

    As the chairs cross exactly half way to the top of the slope, there are exactly the same number of chairs behind (or below) them, i.e. 77 (including chair 15).

    So the total number of chairs is 77 + 77 = 154

11. **C**   Until we answer the question, we can't tell what the variable is. However, we do know that the difference between the evening rate and day rate is equivalent to the variable amount. Once we have that, it becomes easy to answer the question: we just have to look for the option where the difference between the night rate and the evening rate is twice the variable amount (since the variable amount goes from being double to being quadruple). The only option that fits the bill is C, where the fixed fare is £3 and the variable amount £2.

12. **E**   The triangles required to make up the shape in E would not be right-angled but isosceles triangles.

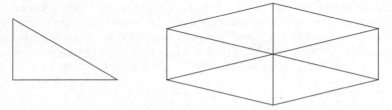

13. **A** The essence of the argument is that whatever God's predetermined purpose for us might be, we would rather do without it so as to be free to choose our own purpose. This rests on the assumption that having the freedom to choose our own purpose is necessarily better than having a predetermined purpose, whatever it might be (A). Note that it also rests on the assumption that having a predetermined purpose is incompatible with having the freedom to choose our own purpose—but that is not one of the answer options. B is an explicit hypothesis or concession, not an underlying assumption of the argument. C and D are assumptions of the counterargument that not to have a pre-determined purpose is, really, not have any purpose at all. E is more of an implicit conclusion than an underlying assumption.

14. **A** The essence of the argument is that, unlike most medical conditions, mental disorders do not have a physical correlate by which they can be defined. As a result, a mental disorder such as schizophrenia is defined according to its supposed symptoms, which themselves are defined according to the concept (or definition) of schizophrenia. Thus, the definitions of schizophrenia and of mental disorders in general are circular (A, E). A is preferable to E because, in the passage, schizophrenia is merely used as an example to illustrate a more general point about all mental disorders. B and C are both false. Most medical conditions are defined by their aetiology or by their pathology, but not mental disorders. This renders mental disorders more difficult to define and recognise. Finally, while D is explicitly stated, it is not the overarching, derivable conclusion of the passage.

15. **B** Distance from JR to Horton is 29 miles.

    Distance from Horton to Churchill is 31 miles.

    Total distance is (29 + 31) 60 miles.

    The doctor gets paid (40 x 0.40) + (20 x 0.30) = 16 + 6 = £22

16. **C** Chrissie takes in (200 x 20) £4,000.

    She must spend: (250 + 1,400 + 150 + (2 x 20 = 40) + (20 x 20 = 400) + (4 x 20 = 80) = £2,320

    To this she must add the cost of the handouts which is: 220 x 0.20 = £44 + 5 = £49 x 20 = £980

    So the total cost of running the course is: 2,320 + 980 = £3,300

    Profit: 4,000 - 3,300 = £700

17. **D** They do overlap: as can be seen, a short elderly man would have a lower expected peak flow rate than a tall young woman.

18. C The passage begins with an imperative statement, 'Don't be envious.' The rest of the passage is provided in support of why you shouldn't be envious. Thus, 'Don't be envious' is the main conclusion of the passage. Don't be misled by the fact that the main conclusion of the passage comes first rather than last. The main conclusion of a passage can come anywhere: at the end, at the beginning, and anywhere in between.

19. C The major premise is a universal affirmative, the minor premise is a universal affirmative, and the conclusion is a particular affirmative.

20. E I have forgotten all men. You are a man. Therefore I have forgotten you. The passage is from *Timon of Athens*, by Shakespeare.

21. D Call the number of 1p coins 'a', which is the same as the number of 5p coins and 10p coins.

1a + 5a + 10a = 192

16a = 192

1 = 192/16 = 12

Alternatively, you could test out each answer option.

22. B You can't tell exactly how many lorries and cars there are on the ferry; however, this doesn't matter as a lorry occupies four times the space of a car and is charged at exactly four times the price.

So, basically, as the deck is full, the ferry operator receives £50 for every 20m² of deck area.

As the deck area is 3,600m², the ferry operator receives 3,600/20 x 50 = 180 x 50 = £9,000

Similarly, since a car carries an average of 2 passengers and a coach carries an average of 8 passengers, there are 180 'units' of 2 people on board the ferry, that is, 360 people.

As they each spend £15, they spend a total of (360 x 15) £5,400.

The amount the ferry operator takes in is therefore (9,000 + 5,400) £14,400.

23. A

24. B   The first part of the passage argues that, for a variety of reasons, people in modern societies are more likely to interpret their distress in terms of depression (A). Building upon this, the second part of the passage further argues that this has gone too far, and that the concept of depression as a mental disorder has been overextended to include all manner of human suffering (B). D is only a part of that argument. E is in keeping with the spirit of the passage, but is a step too far. Similarly, though highly plausible, there is nothing in the text that enables us to conclude that people in modern societies find it easier to think of their problems in terms of a mental disorder (C). But in any case, this would not constitute the main conclusion of the passage.

25. D   The argument is essentially that studying for an MBA is no longer the best use of your time and resources. All five propositions strengthen the argument. But whereas A, B, C, and E merely flesh out the premise that an MBA is not or no longer such a good proposition, D supports the conclusion that you should instead try an internship or start your own business.

26. B   The principal flaw in the argument is that it assumes that schizophrenia-sufferers generally or invariably present a high risk to others. However, the vast majority of schizophrenia-sufferers are no more likely to be violent than the average person.

27. D   If the Roystons bought just day entry fees, they would pay: 40 x (4.50 + 4.50 + 3.00 + 3.00 = £15) = £600

If they bought annual passes, they would pay: £42 + £42 + £28 + £28 = £140

So they would save: 600 - 140 = £460

28. B   The balance between the winemaker and the grower is (2,600 - 2,200) £400, owed by the winemaker to the grower.

The balance between the winemaker and the chemist is (600 - 300) £300 owed by the chemist to the winemaker.

The balance between the grower and the chemist is £600, owed by the grower to the chemist.

So, the winemaker owes £400 to the grower, the grower £600 to the chemist, and the chemist £300 to the winemaker.

Since each party will be giving £300 to one of the other two parties, and receiving £300 from the other, they do not gain or lose any of that money. Thus, the transfer of the extra £300 in each sum could be seen as redundant.

Beyond that, the winemaker owes £100 to the grower, and the grower £300 to the chemist.

So the winemaker should pay the grower £100, and the grower should pay the chemist £300.

29. D First of all, the cost per person will *fall*, eliminating A.

The cost per person for one person is: 18 + 4 = £22

The cost per person for two people is: (22 + 4) £26/2 = £13

The cost per person for three people is: (26 + 4) £30/3 = £10

And so on.

B is similar to D, but starts at £18 rather than £22. But, of course, you can't have zero people in the boat!

30. C The passage states that NIDDM is closely associated with obesity, but does not state or assume that NIDDM is caused by obesity (A). Other factors are also involved in the aetiology (causation) of NIDDM, for example, genetic predisposition. This means that there could be significant regional variations in the prevalence of NIDDM in the population group under study (C). There may also be significant variations in the numbers of people with a BMI greater than 30 (B), but these variations are controlled for by the study, which expresses its findings in terms of prescription rates rather than the absolute number of prescriptions. Be careful to read through all the options, without which you might have been tempted to select B! The pharmaceutical company very likely has a vested interested in publishing the study (E), but, whereas this might touch upon the findings, it does not touch upon the argument as such. Similarly, the argument does not fall apart if the drug is only somewhat more effective than its alternatives (D).

31. D It may be true that physicists are not representative of academics as a whole (A), but the information in the passage does not warrant such a conclusion. B and C are explicitly stated in the passage: unlike D, they are not a derived conclusion. Whereas B and C describe the results of the study, D describes the conclusion that can be drawn or derived from those results, namely, that, as far as physics is concerned, elite universities do not add value to output. It is, however, a step too far to conclude that authorities should not concentrate physics research into fewer, more elite institutions (E).

32. E The argument is that the Council wasted money on the exercise stations because current visitors to the arboretum do not like them. However, the Council's aim was not to please current visitors, but to attract more visitors. This aim will be achieved if the exercise stations attract more visitors than they put off (E). The second best answer is C, but E is a complete, and therefore better, statement of the flaw in the argument. A does not touch directly upon the argument. With B, the Council could still have failed to attract new visitors and thereby wasted money. D rather supports the argument; it is not a flaw.

33. B Tom's current mixture consists of (30 x 500/100) 150kg sand and (500 – 150) 350kg loam.

So he needs to have 350kg of sand if the mixture is to consist of 50% sand.

For that, he needs to add (350 – 150) 200kg of sand to the mixture.

34. E Area of wall (length x height)/area of a roll of wallpaper

Make sure to convert 60cm into metres!

35. D Calculate the amount of petrol used for each leg of the journey by dividing the distance covered by 100 and multiplying by the fuel consumption (divide by 100 because fuel consumption is expressed in 1/100m). Don't forget to multiply by 2 to account for the return journey. Then sum up the petrol used for each leg of the journey and multiply by the cost of petrol. You don't need to calculate this exactly; you should be able to see that the answer will be just short of £12.

Urban roads: (5/100 x 10) x 2 = 1l

Country roads: (20/100 x 12) x 2 = 4.8l

Motorway: (30/100 x 15) x 2 = 9l

Total = 14.8l

Cost of fuel = 14.8 x £0.80 = £11.84

36. C The argument is that, because households are borrowing more and devoting more pay to mortgage repayments, they have less money to spend on consumption: this hurts firms and workers and reduces investment, which lowers GDP now and in the future. Thus, a high level of household indebtedness poses a risk to the economy (C). All the other answer options are parts of the argument rather than its main conclusion.

37. E Of course, people do not necessarily need to work hard to start a successful business: they might, for example, have had such a brilliant idea that it just takes off by itself (B, D). But even if people do need to work hard to start a successful business, working hard is not the only condition required for the success of a business. Other factors may also be involved, such as an inspired idea, adequate seed capital, and luck (C, A). Therefore, while working hard may be a necessary condition for the success of a business, it is not a sufficient condition (E). The argument itself turns more on E than on B.

38. B The argument is, in essence, that 'mental disorder' is difficult to define because (1) mental disorders lie on a continuum of human experience, and (2) they may not map onto any real or distinct disease entities… 'Furthermore' (B) introduces additional supporting information. A and D introduce contrast. C introduces qualification. E introduces comparison.

39. C Let 'a' be the number of 20p stamps and '3a' the number of 50p stamps.

(a x 0.2) + (3a x 0.5) = 10.20

0.2a + 1.5a = 10.20

1.7a = 10.20

10.2/1.7 = a = 6

The total number of stamps is (a + 3a) 4a i.e. 24.

Alternatively, you can work backwards and test out each option.

40. B 13 rolls of wallpaper x £25 each = £325 - 20% trade discount (£65) = £260

2 pots of glue x £6 = £12 - 20% trade discount (£2.40) = £9.60

8 hours x 15 = £120 + 20% VAT (£24) = £144

Total = 260 + 9.60 + 144 = £413.60

41. B

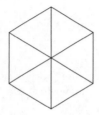

42. E The argument is that train operators could ease overcrowding and offer a better service by doing away with First Class and converting First Class carriages to standard class. But if the revenue raised by First Class helps to fund standard class carriages, then doing away with First Class could well result in fewer standard class carriages and a poorer service. E and B make similar points, but B does not specify that the extra revenue funds standard class carriages. A, C, and D cannot directly undermine the argument.

43. E Europeans are more likely to either abstain from voting (B) or vote for an anti-European party (C). Therefore, the European Union is deeply unpopular (E).

44. C The principle being highlighted is the so-called Principle of Subsidiarity, which states that a matter ought to be handled by the smallest, lowest, or least centralised authority capable of addressing that matter effectively. Some of the benefits of subsidiarity include empowering people; increasing their political participation; and, by generating diverse solutions to common problems, avoiding systemic failures.

45. D   Value of commission = 4,600 – 1,200 = £3,400

This amounts to 2% of sales.

Therefore total sales = (100/2) x 3,400 = £170,000

46. D   It can be very helpful to sketch the initial diagram on a piece of paper, which you can then rotate in various directions and compare to the answer options. Focus on the spatial relationship between the four visible symbols and take it from there.

47. A   We know that the buildings in the row to the left of Greg (and in front of Priya) are never higher than the equivalent of three boxes. We also know that there is only one building in that row, in the middle of the row. Therefore, that one building (which is facing Priya) has to be at least three boxes high. This means that Priya's view of that row cannot be of fewer than three boxes.

48. B   The basic form of the argument is: X depends on Y. No Y. Therefore, no X.

49. A   In essence, the argument is that wage rises will increase productivity because firms will invest more in machines and software. This assumes that the firms want to control their costs as much as possible, and will therefore do whatever costs them less. It is true that low wages are good for employment (B): but while so much can be inferred from the passage, it is not an underlying assumption of the argument. Similarly, one might infer that machines and software cannot replace high-skilled work (C), but the argument hardly turns around this point. D on the other hand is simply wrong: the passage implies that workers' productivity increases as a result of *higher* investment. Finally, the argument explicitly assumes that, while economists can be wrong (E), in this case, they are right. In other words, that economists are always right is not an underlying assumption of the argument.

50. E   The passage contains two propositions, which must be read together to be fully understood. The first proposition, contained in the first sentence, is that we are carried around by our unconscious will (the blind giant)—and so 'mostly driven by unconscious forces' (E). The second proposition, contained in the second sentence, is that our conscious intellect may not be entirely or even mostly cognizant of our unconscious will. We may think that our intellect is in charge, but this is merely a 'delusion' (making D false). The rest of the passage is an example to illustrate these two propositions. The blind giant of will is anything but powerless (making B false), while, of course, the lame man represents our conscious intellect (making A false). Finally, while the passage does state that Schopenhauer anticipates Freud, one is not entitled to conclude that he actually inspired the work of Freud (C). For example, Freud may never have read, or even heard about, Schopenhauer.

Good luck!

If you have any thoughts for improving this book, please email them to neel@neelburton.com.